Meal Planning for Beginners:

The Healthy Meal Prep Cookbook with 80+ Quick and Easy Recipes, Weekly Plans and Ready-to-Go Meals

Copyright © 2019 Thomas Teselli
All rights reserved

Disclaimer

The information in this book is for informational purposes only. While every effort has been made to provide proper nutritional information, this book is not meant to be a replacement for medical advice. Please speak to your primary care physician before starting any new diet or exercise program.

TABLE OF CONTENTS

Introduction V
Chapter 1: What Are Macronutrients? 1
    Macros: The Building Blocks of Food 2
    A Closer Look at Macronutrients 2
    Calorie Counting vs. Macro Counting 6
    Putting This Information to Use 8
    Using Food Labels: Measures and Weights 11
    How Do Carb/Protein/Fat Work in the Body? 14
    Setting Weight Goals 15

Chapter 2: Prepping for Success 16
    Spring Clean-Out! 16
    Essential Kitchen Tools 17
    The Mediterranean Pantry 18
    Cooking and Prepping Terms & Techniques 19
    Guide to Notations 21

Chapter 3: Meal Planning 22
    Shopping Tips 22
    What Is a Meal Plan? 22
    21-Day Meal Plan 30

Chapter 4: Altering the Meal Plan to Fit Your Goals 45
Chapter 5: Breakfast 46
Chapter 6: Lunch Break 69
Chapter 7: Dinner 107
Chapter 8: Desserts 140
Chapter 9: Snacks and Sides 155

Chapter 10: Shopping Guide and Food List 186
   Foods to Eat: 186
   Pantry List: 186
   Fresh List: 187

Chapter 11: Charting Your Success 188
   Weight/Macro Chart 188
   Set Up Your Goal 188
   Make Your Meal Plan 189
   Exercise Chart 190
   Recipe Macro/Calorie Table 191
   Online Resources 197

Conclusion 199

Introduction

Congratulations on downloading *Meal Planning for Beginners*, and thank you for doing so. *Meal Planning for Beginners* builds on the information provided in the companion book *The Complete Mediterranean Diet for Beginners*.

The following chapters will discuss the basics of meal planning and preparation. Soon, you will begin to enjoy healthy, delicious food prepared in your own home. Cook for your friends with confidence, and share your knowledge and skill of healthy cooking. Also, all of the recipes in this book have the macro grams figured to make building your own unique diet a snap.

You will also learn a different way of looking at calories. Counting macros vs. counting calories first became popular among weightlifters. The word "macros" refers to the macronutrients that make up our food. But more about that later. What's important is that this information will allow you to take control of the food you eat. You have the power to decide how you will fuel your body and with what.

The recipes in this book will follow the Mediterranean diet, which is rich in fresh fruits, vegetables, lean meats, seafood, whole grains, nuts, and olive oil. Recipes use Standard (imperial) measurements rather than metric. And, unless otherwise stated, all ingredients are fresh—no powdered garlic, no lemon juice out of a jar. They are just not as flavorful and do not save money.

Below is an outline of information and tools to help you reach your health goal:

- Introduction to macronutrients (often referred to as macros)
- Learning to count macros instead of simply counting calories
- Essential tools you will need to prepare and cook your meals
- Food selection and preparation
- Tips and techniques for the kitchen
- Meal planning for 21 days of delicious meals
- How to modify meals or recipes to help you reach your goals
- Over 80+ recipes with nutritional information
- Shopping guide and food list
- Tools to help you reach your goals

By cooking one or two meals a day, you will begin saving money, lose some weight, and maybe even develop a lifelong habit of good eating. Reviewing the ingredients in these recipes will help you make better choices when eating out.

There are plenty of books on this subject on the market; thanks again for choosing this one! Every effort was made to ensure it is full of as much useful information as possible. Please enjoy!

Chapter 1: What Are Macronutrients?

Remember the old food pyramid where the large, sturdy base was made up of bread, cereal, and other carbohydrates, six to eleven servings per day? The next level contained vegetables with three to five servings and fruits with two to four servings. Then, higher up but with smaller servings required are the dairy, meat, egg, nuts, and beans with two to three servings. This was all crowned by fats, oils, and sweets at the tip top. There are no serving suggestions but a warning that said: "USE SPARINGLY."

These guidelines sounded reasonable and made sense with what we knew about the body's use of nutrition. But, what the food pyramid didn't take into account is that most foods contain some carbs, protein, and fat. Our bodies need a balance of these nutrients to function efficiently by burning unwanted fat but not running out of energy.

Because of that first introduction to the basic food groups, there is a tendency to think of bread as strictly carbohydrate. Vegetables, fruits, and foods at the same level are thought of as health food. In other words, you can eat them as much as you want, while most types of meat, dairy, eggs, and nuts are good-for-you protein. On top of the pyramid is fat. "So, who eats a stick of butter? I shouldn't have a problem with fat!"

Fortunately, food science and our understanding of how we break down the components of food have come a long way since the first attempt to help people eat healthily. The old version of the food pyramid laid the groundwork for a variety of new views. Diets such as Paleo, Atkins, Keto, and others are formulated around increasing or decreasing the intake of carbs, proteins, and fats.

It turns out that those three main elements of carbohydrates, proteins, and fats are the three major nutrients contained in the food we eat. *They are called macronutrients* or macros for short.

Macros: The Building Blocks of Food

We have to re-learn the way we think of food. Instead of thinking of bread as a carb, an apple as "health food," an egg as protein, or walnut as fat, we look at the percentage of all three macros in the food. What percentage of carbs, protein, and fat do the bread, apple, egg, and walnut contain?

It sounds complicated, but it really isn't. The percentages are conveniently contained on the product's nutrition label. For whole foods such as avocado or spaghetti squash, there are online nutrient calculators that you can use to figure the percentage spread.

Are you feeling overwhelmed? Don't be. By the time you finish these first few chapters, you will be a pro at figuring your macro percentages needed to reach your goals. You will also have the tools you need to find the proper food to fuel your body.

A Closer Look at Macronutrients

1. Carbohydrates:

You have probably heard about simple and complex carbohydrates. Here is a definition refresher.

Simple carbs break down fast and are absorbed quickly into the bloodstream. Some foods that are considered simple carbs are: *refined sugar, fruit juice, candy, honey, white potatoes, white rice, refined white flour, alcohol, syrups, and sodas.*

Complex carbs, on the other hand, are released slowly in the bloodstream over some time to help sustain your body's energy. Some foods that are considered complex carbs are: quinoa, brown rice, beans, lentils, oatmeal, and peas.

Are you familiar with the term sugar rush? That's what happens when your energy slumps, and you feel tired, so you eat a simple carb (say, a chocolate bar) to give you quick energy. Unfortunately, this quick fix of energy burns out as fast as it peaks. Then, you experience a sugar crash, which leaves you feeling worse than before.

Layering complex carbs with simple carbs is a better use of this nutritional building block. Cyclist will carbo-load with whole grains and other complex carbs several days before a big ride so that they have an extra store of energy (glycogen) in the muscles and liver. This prevents the athlete from running out of energy before finishing the race.

During the race, the athlete can consume some simple carbs to give him or her an extra boost of energy. This is not harmful because the athlete is burning up calories at an amazing rate.

For those of us sitting and watching the race, we don't need that sugary drink or sweet snack. Unfortunately, we are not burning many calories as we cheer on the riders.

Beware of cutting too many carbs out of your diet. If the body does not have enough carbohydrate to convert into glucose, it will start using protein and fat to do this process. This method of creating glucose has a waste product called ketones that build up in the body, causing the kidneys to work extra hard to clear out the waste.

The fiber in carbohydrates plays an important role in the health and welfare of your body. Keeping your bowel movements regular is what fiber is best known for, but dietary fiber appears to have a much more important role. High-fiber diets appear to lower risk of heart disease, high blood pressure, diabetes, and obesity.

2. Protein:

Protein is not stored in the body but is found in almost every part of the body, nails, hair, skin, bone, muscle, and tissue.

Proteins are made up of more than twenty different amino acids, nine of which are essential and must come from the food you eat. The body gets these amino acids in one of two ways: building them from scratch or modifying others. Foods called *high-quality proteins* such as dairy products, meat, and eggs, have all the essential amino acids that the body requires.

Compare red meat, ham steak, grilled salmon, chicken, and lentils/beans. Take into account fat and salt content. You will find that protein from dairy (whey), grilled fish, some chicken and lentils/beans are the best option to lower saturated fats and sodium.

And, you can do the environment some good by cutting down on red meat as the methane gas created by all those cows contributes to the greenhouse effect. Greenhouse gas emissions by cattle as a natural part of their digestive process and how we deal with the manure help contribute to the buildup of greenhouse gases in our atmosphere.

3. Fat:

Saturated Fats — Animal fats such as lard (bacon fat) and dairy fats (butter, cheese) and anything hard at room temperature contains saturated fat. You also need to steer clear of some tropical oils such as palm and palm kernel and coconut.

Trans Fats — Stay away from these manufactured fats that are created by hydrogenating oils (forcing extra hydrogen atoms onto a fat chain hardens the oils). If you see partially hydrogenated oil on the food label, that is code for trans fats. Try to avoid eating this product.

Unsaturated Fats:

Monounsaturated fats — Sources of monounsaturated fats are avocados, nuts, seeds, and olives. Also, oils, peanut, canola, and olive oils are good sources of this fat.

Polyunsaturated fats — These include omega-3 fatty acids, walnuts, ground flaxseed, tofu and soybeans, canola, soybean, and walnut oils. Bluefish, herring, lake trout, mackerel, salmon, sardines, and tuna are also sources of polyunsaturated fats.

Omega-6 fatty acids — These include sunflower seeds, Brazil nuts, pecans, and pine nuts. Cooking oils include corn, sunflower, safflower, and sesame oils.

Calorie Counting vs. Macro Counting

What is the difference between counting calories and counting macros? When we count calories, we are counting the number of calories (energy) we consume from the food regardless of the nutrient source. When counting macros, we count the calories consumed from each of the nutrients.

This is the calculation you need to remember to find out where your calories come from:

- One gram of carbs = 4 calories
- One gram of protein = 4 calories
- One gram of fat = 9 calories

The basic ratio your body needs per day is 30% carbs, 40% protein, and 30% fat. Now, this can change depending on your personal health goals that you have set up with your physician.

For example, the average slice of whole grain with seed bread has about 120 calories per slice listed on the food label. So that's 120 calories used up from our daily allotted amount. But in terms of macros we read: carbs 22g, protein 5g, and fats 2g.

Using our calories per gram formula above, we do the following:

- 22g of carbs * 4 calories = 88 calories from carbs
- 5g of protein * 4 calories = 20 calories from protein
- 2 grams of fat * 9 calories = 18 calories from fat

- Giving: 88 + 20 + 18 = 126 calories per slice.

Again, using an online fitness tool with a built-in nutrition calculator makes tracking your intake much easier. For your convenience, there is a page at the back of the book for manual tracking to get you started and a list of sites that provide online calculators.

Male: 55, 5' 11", current weight 185, goal weight 170. Lightly active (moderate exercise by sedentary job). This person wants to lose fifteen pounds.

Using the online Macronutrient Calculator from *www.bodybuilding.com*, the daily macros needed to lose weight at a moderate pace would be 168 g carbs, 168 g protein, and 37 g fats per day. Taking this one step further:

- 168g * 4c = 672 carbs
- 168g * 4c = 672 protein
- 37g * 9c = 333 fat
- Giving: 672+672+333= 1677 calories per day

Using the online calorie calculator from *www.freedieting.com*, I find that: maintenance is 2335 cals per day, fat loss is 1868 cals per day, and extreme fat loss is 1480 cals per day.

Because we do not know exactly how these sites are creating their numbers, talk to your doctor in order to find out what calories per day is best for your weight goal.

Using calories of 1868 per day in the macro calculator, the macro ratio comes to 40% carbs,

30% protein, and 30% fat.

Grams per day = 186g carbs, 140g protein, and 62g fat.

- 186g * 4c = 744 carb
- 140g * 4c = 560 protein
- 62g * 9c = 558
- Giving: 744+560+558 = 1862 cals per day.

Putting This Information to Use

Sex: M

Weight: 190

Height: 5' 11"

Exercise: 3 times a week, 30 minutes

Job: Sedentary

Goal Weight: 170, loss of 20 lbs

Maintain: 2138 calories

Moderate Fat Loss: 1710 calories

Extreme Fat Loss: 1520 calories

Sex: F

Weight: 170

Height: 5' 4"

Exercise: 3 times a week, 30 minutes

Job: Sedentary

Goal Weight: 150, loss of 20 lbs

Maintain: 1860 calories

Moderate Fat Loss: 1488 calories

Extreme Fat Loss: 1360 calories

Using several well-established restaurants and their online nutritional information, I came up with an example of what might be a typical meal plan for the average American.

MEAL PLANNING FOR BEGINNERS

Breakfast	Table 1	gCarbs	gProt	gFat	cCarbs	cProt	cFat	Calories
	2 Scrambled	2	15	17	8	60	153	221
	Whole Grain Toast with butter, jam	58	7	11	232	28	99	359
	Hash Browns	19	2	14	76	8	126	210
	Bacon, 2 slices	1	7	7	4	28	63	95
Lunch	SW Chicken Club	43	29	29	172	116	261	549
Dinner	Meatloaf with mashed potatoes and broccoli	92	44	42	368	176	378	922
Daily Totals		**215**	**104**	**120**	**860**	**416**	**1080**	**2356**

As you can see in Table 1, one size does not fit all. Both male and female are over the maintenance range, but the female is way over. This may be part of the reason that women have a bigger struggle with weight loss. Portions are geared toward larger bodies with bigger appetites. Combine large portions of high fat and carb options with our eating on-the-fly American lifestyle, and you have a recipe for obesity.

Look for ways you can change your meal to better fit your new habits. Order the eggs poached or basted (cooked in water or steamed). Eat one slice of toast and have it dry (no butter or jam). Or, make sure you order the toast dry so that you can control how much fat and sugar you add. Skip the hash browns altogether, or see if they have a fresh fruit option. Bacon was a better choice than sausage, so no change is needed.

The easiest change for lunch and supper is to cut the order in half. Order half a sub, or better yet, make it veggie with grilled chicken, vinegar only, and no oil. With the dinner, ask for a to-go box, and put half aside for lunch tomorrow. You can look at the grid above to see how much you save by cutting things in half and leaving off the extras.

Let's look at some more information that needs to be taken into account when trying to improve our eating habits.

Using Food Labels: Measures and Weights

One of the best laws our government ever passed for the people of the United States is Public Law 101-535, which is the Nutrition Labeling and Education Act (NLEA).

President George H. W. Bush signed the act into law on November 8, 1990.

This law gives the FDA (Food and Drug Administration) authority to require nutrition labels on almost everything we eat. Over the past 30 years, the label contents have been enhanced to include valuable information for consumers.

Let's take a look at a label to see what information is included.

Nutrition Facts

Serving Size 1 cup (228g)
Servings Per Container 2 ← Start here

Amount Per Serving

Calories 250   Calories from Fat 110 ← Check calories

                                    % Daily Value* ← Quick guide to % DV

Total Fat 12g	18%
Saturated Fat 3g	15%
Trans Fat 3g	
Cholesterol 30mg	10%
Sodium 470mg	20%
Potassium 700mg	20%
Total Carbohydrate 31g	10%
Dietary Fiber 0g	0%
Sugars 5g	
Protein 5g	
Vitamin A	4%
Vitamin C	2%
Calcium	20%
Iron	4%

- 5% or less is low
- 20% or more is high ← (Total Fat, Saturated Fat, Trans Fat)
- Limit these ← (Cholesterol, Sodium)
- Get enough of these ← (Potassium, Total Carbohydrate, Dietary Fiber, Sugars, Protein)
- Footnote ← (Iron)

* Percent Daily Values are based on a 2,000 calorie diet. Your Daily Values may be higher or lower depending on your calorie needs.

	Calories:	2,000	2,500
Total Fat	Less than	65g	80g
Sat Fat	Less than	20g	25g
Cholesterol	Less than	300mg	300mg
Sodium	Less than	2,400mg	2,400mg
Total Carbohydrate		300g	375g
Dietary Fiber		25g	30g

Using a bread label for this example, **Nutrition Facts** heads the familiar column of information.

First up is the **Serving Size** listed in standard units, followed by metric units, and then **Servings Per Container**. Pay attention to serving size. Some bread labels are 1 slice, some 2 slices. You can torpedo all your hard work if you think you are logging macros for 2 slices when it was actually 1 slice serving.

Serving information is always followed by **Calories** per serving and **Calories from Fat**. Try to steer clear of food that has more than 50% of calories from fat. One exception would be avocado, which is high in fat but no saturated or trans fats. This is an example of a food that has fats necessary for hormone production and cell maintenance.

In the next block of the label, we find the nutrients, including the macros. The nutrients are listed in metric along with the percentage based on the daily requirement of 2000 calories. Here, you will find **Total Fat** broken down by **Saturated Fat** and **Trans Fat**. **Cholesterol, Sodium, Potassium** are listed next and are especially important to people with diabetes, high blood pressure, and other life-threatening diseases. **Total Carbohydrates** is broken down into **Dietary Fiber** and **Sugars**. Items high in dietary fiber are a much better choice than those with high sugar numbers (sometimes added) and little or no dietary fiber. The last item in the nutrients is **Protein**.

The next block of the label list **trace vitamins and minerals** contained in the product. These listings come in handy when you are trying to increase or limit a certain vitamin or mineral. For example, if you are on a medication that requires a low vitamin K diet, this is the place on the label you would check for the percentage of daily requirements of vitamin K this serving of food fulfills.

The final block of the label is an explanation of the minimum daily requirements based on a 2000 calorie diet and sometimes, a 2500 calorie diet.

Don't forget to check the *ingredients list* that usually follows the nutrition label. If you are purchasing something that claims to be made with chicken, is chicken the first ingredient? If not, do you really want to eat that product?

Also, if the ingredients list contains "partially hydrogenated ...," skip this item. That means that the product contains trans fats, and you do not want to add those to your diet.

How Do Carb/Protein/Fat Work in the Body?

Macronutrients are the three building blocks of food that your body need to thrive, but how do carbs, protein, and fats work to fuel your body?

Carbohydrates — Both simple and complex carbs are converted into energy by the body in the form of glucose, the main source of energy for the body. Though, as we saw above, complex carbs do a better job of giving us a steady flow of energy.

Carbs also benefit the body in other ways. The fiber found in many carbs helps clean our bowels and appear to help with some health issues, such as reducing high blood pressure, diabetes, and obesity.

Protein — Made of components called amino acids, protein is in charge of growth and tissue repair. A quick reminder: there are 20 different amino acids. Eleven of these, we produce with our bodies, and nine essentials must be obtained from the food we eat.

Fat — The macronutrient fat has its share of important functions. We think of it mainly as a means of storing excess energy—in the form of fat. But, it is also instrumental in absorbing the fat-soluble vitamins (A, D, E and K), which are used in the production of some hormones and help with maintaining cell structures.

Setting Weight Goals

This is where meal planning really helps. As you can see above, the amount of food and what the meal consists of are extremely important.

To give meal planning a chance, you need to set up your food intake to match the outcome desired. Take your weight prior to starting the three weeks. Leave the scales alone during your first three weeks on the plan, then check the results. I'm guessing you really won't be surprised, because your clothes will fit better or feel a bit loose, and you'll be feeling better.

Using the tools you have been given, work up your meal plan based on your weight loss goals. Then, make an appointment with your doctor to have him or her review the plan with you.

Chapter 2: Prepping for Success

Spring Clean-Out!

You want this change to happen. You want to save money and control your weight. So let's start with a clean, out-with-the-old to make room for the new.

Take inventory of your refrigerator and your pantry. After reading through the recipes and ingredients, you may find many items in your kitchen that are not part of the Mediterranean diet.

Toss them out, or give them away even if you just bought them. Let it go. If it's not helping you reach your goal of having better health or a better-looking you. Let it go.

If there are others in the household, it is important to get them on board and excited about what you are planning to accomplish. There are nights when others may want a meal that is so far off the grid that you don't think of it as food anymore.

Let it go. Let them eat what they want, but talk about it the next day. I'm willing to bet they will tell you it didn't sit well with their digestive system, and they didn't feel good the next day.

Or, if it's something fun but high in fat, such as pizza, have a slice with a big salad and lots of water. It's okay to have off-plan days as long as you plan for it!

Essential Kitchen Tools

If these items aren't already in your cabinets, check out garage sales, estate sales, and thrift shops before going to the department store. You can probably get most of these items for a quarter of what you would spend in the department store.

- Saucepans with lid - 1.5 qt. and 3 qt.
- Stockpot with lid - 6 qt.
- Nonstick skillet - 9.5" and 12"
- Cast iron skillet - at least 12"
- Set of stainless mixing bowls (s, m, l)
- Pyrex bakeware - 9x13 pan, large pie dish
- Stainless bakeware - 9x9, 9x13, 9" pie pan
- Baking or cookie sheet
- Vegetable knife (12" wedge shape blade)
- Paring knife (3" blade)
- Large slotted spoon
- Ladle
- Meat fork (sturdier than a regular fork)
- Spatula (variety of metal and rubber)
- Measuring spoons
- Measuring cups (1 c. and 2c.)
- Wisk
- Zester (tiny grater)
- Peppermill
- Meat thermometer
- Food processor
- Shrimp deveiner
- Microwave oven

The Mediterranean Pantry

Keeping your pantry stocked with the basics cuts down on frustration. There is nothing worse than planning to make your favorite dish then remembering you are out of something essential just as you are reaching for it.

Basic Items

- Olive oil, safflower oil, raw coconut oil, and butter
- Skim milk, feta cheese, and non-homogenized yogurt
- Whole wheat flour, unbleached white
- Sugar, honey, maple syrup, and stevia (if you want to cut down on refined sugar)
- Soy sauce and Worcestershire sauce
- Sea salt and black peppercorns
- Quinoa, couscous, and brown rice
- Garlic and yellow onions
- Green olives and Greek olives
- Canned: garbanzo beans and beets
- Dried or ground: cumin, thyme, oregano, cinnamon, paprika, red pepper flakes, chili powder, and dill weed
- Baking powder and baking soda
- Mayonnaise and mustard (yellow, stone ground, Dijon)

Advanced Items

- Coriander, mustard seeds, bay leaf, curry, whole nutmegs, cardamom, ground mustard, turmeric, and white peppercorns
- Capers
- Almond flour, buckwheat, ground flax seed, and wheat germ

Cooking and Prepping Terms & Techniques

- **Poaching** - Protein cooked in liquid.
- **Blanching** - Process to trap nutrients in vegetables, kill bacteria, and lock in color. It is also a method of popping skins off of nuts.
- **Yogurt cheese** - non-homogenized yogurt with the whey drained out.
- **Sweating** - Cooking vegetables (usually onions and garlic) over a low heat with the lid on until translucent and limp.
- **Caramelizing** - Vegetables, cooked at low heat in a little fat for a long time so that the natural sugars in the vegetables brown as they cook.
- **Sauté** - A quick fry in very little fat.
- **Simmer** - Liquid that stays just below boiling point.
- **Braising** - A technique that uses quick hot, dry heat followed by long low heat and liquid. Pot roast is made by braising. The roast is first seared on all sides over high heat with oil only. Then the heat is reduced, and liquid is added as the roast cooks slowly to break down connective fibers (collagen) that make the meat tough.
- **Chopping basil** - I find basil has a better taste if not handled too much. A simple chop, no mincing. The exception is when making pesto.
- **Faster boiling** - Use your lids. The heat gets trapped, and the water warms faster.
- **Buttermilk substitutions:**
  Buttermilk powder: Add 1/4 cup buttermilk powder to the 1 cup of the dry mix along with 1 large egg and 1 cup water or milk.
  Yogurt: Substitute Greek-style or standard plain yogurt for the buttermilk, thinning batter to the desired consistency as necessary.
  Dairy milk or plant-based milk: Mix 1 tablespoon white or apple cider vinegar or lemon juice, with enough milk to measure 1 cup; mix thoroughly and let rest for 5 minutes before using.

- **Roasting Peppers** - The goal is to blister the skin of the pepper without burning the flesh. This can be done in several ways. If you only have one or two to roast, you can hold them over the gas flame of your range.
  If you have an electric stove or quite a few peppers to roast, it's easiest to use the broiler. As the side toward the heat starts to blister and blacken, turn pepper to the other side. Continue to watch and rotate so that the pepper does not burn all the way through. Cool

peppers in a paper bag to help sweat loose the skins.

- **Substitute for sun-dried tomatoes** - In a slow oven (250 degrees), place a baking sheet fit with parchment paper and cover with tomato halves (grape or plum) drizzled with olive oil. Cook for 60-90 minutes until tomatoes have reduced in size, by about half.
- **Colanders** - Always have a bowl or saucepan on hand to side under these, or else you will have liquid everywhere, and sometimes it's very hot.
- **Silverskin** - Tendon that adheres to the meat is called silverskin. To remove, slide a sharp paring knife underneath the length of the tendon.
- **Hand washing** - You should constantly be rinsing or washing your hands. Before you start cooking, after handling raw meat, after you handle your phone, if you grab the remote to change the channel on the TV or dial on the radio—WASH YOUR HANDS.
- **Cross-contamination** - If a tool, pan, plate, etc. have come in contact with raw meat, do not reuse it without washing it in soap and hot water. BBQ for friends? Don't set the meat tray to one side while you cook the chicken so you can use the same tray to take it back inside. You could make everyone very sick.
- **Marinades** - I'm seeing a disturbing trend in recipes where cooks instruct the readers to reserve marinade that has already come in contact with the raw protein. NEVER reuse marinade; it contains bacteria from the raw protein that can make you very sick. Save some marinade aside when you first make it, before soaking the meat.
- **Olive Oil** - To save on space, I have abbreviated extra-virgin olive oil to read as "olive oil" or "evoo." Please do your research and get a good quality olive oil.
- **Garlic** - The easiest way to peel a clove of garlic is to crush it under the broad side of the veggie knife. You can do this with a paring knife, but the clove might shoot out from under the blade. How do I know this? Smashing it in this manner also releases the juice and oils. Now, you are ready to cut off the hard end, and slice, chop, or mince.

Guide to Notations

- qt = quart
- pt = pint
- c = cup
- tea = teaspoon
- T = tablespoon
- lbs = pounds
- g = grams
- .3 = 1/3
- .66 = 2/3
- .25 = 1/4
- .5 = 1/2
- .75 = 3/4

Chapter 3: Meal Planning

Shopping Tips

- **Buy organic** if you possibly can
- **Fresh fish** - Look for bright, clear, and bulging eyes. If they look sunken and cloudy, the fish is probably old. Don't buy it. With the exception of deep-sea fish, such as salmon, which is flash frozen at the catch, you want to purchase fish with the head still attached so you can see that it is fresh.
- **Fleshy fruits** - Nectarines, peaches, pears, avocado, and the like should have a wonderful aroma when you gently squeeze them. They should not be rock hard or mushy. Apples should be hard and crisp. Melons should also smell sweet, and you may learn the art of thumping melons to determine if they are ripe. It's a good, dense thump or thud. If it sounds hollow, the melon is probably not ripe.
- **Lemons/limes** - I find that the thinner and smoother the skin feels, the more juice there is, which is especially true for limes.
- **Meats and poultry** – Meat should look pink and plump. There should be no discoloration (tinge of brown, green) to the meat. Chicken that has a grey, sallow look is getting old.

What Is a Meal Plan?

A meal plan is a means to keep your eating on track with your goals. There are a few variables to keep in mind. How much time do you have to prepare the meals? What keeps best in the refrigerator at work, if you work? How much can you make ahead of time, say Sunday afternoon, which will last the entire week?

Let's look at this first meal plan. With the exception of the breakfast (which takes about 5 minutes to make) and dinner (which is best served warm out of the oven), these may be made ahead of time and packed for work.

MEAL PLANNING FOR BEGINNERS

Table 2	Carbs	Protein	Fat	Totals
Breakfast	Basted Egg with Smoked Salmon on Toast			
grams	28	13	19	
calories	112	52	171	335
Lunch	Citrus Pesto Chicken Salad			
grams	4	25	5	
calories	16	100	45	161
	Lemon Mustard Dressing			
grams	1	0	2	
calories	4	0	18	22
snack	Jumpin' Quinoa Munch Bars			
grams	12	2	4	
calories	48	8	36	92
dinner	Baked Greek Salmon in a Pouch			
grams	9	40	28	
calories	36	160	252	448
	Savory Herb Roasted Potatoes			
grams	23	3	4	
calories	92	12	36	140
	Side Salad			
grams	3	1	0.5	
calories	12	4	4.5	20.5
	Red Wine Vinaigrette			
grams	0.5	0	3	
calories	2	0	27	29
snack	Evening Pick-Me-Up			
grams	6	12	21	
calories	24	48	189	261
Total G	86.5	96	86.5	
Total C	346	384	778.5	1508.5

	Carbs	Protein	Fat
GRAMS per day	93g	148g	57g
GRAMS per meal	18.6g	29.6g	11.4g
CALORIES per day	372 cals	595 cals	521 cals

Female, age: 55, weight: 170 lbs, height: 5' 4"

Goal: Lose 20 lbs at a moderate pace

Information from www.freedieting.com

Macro Ratio: 25% carbs, 40% prot, 35% fat

Calories for fat loss: 1488

Calories for extreme fat loss: 1360

Grams per day	93g	148g	57g
	under	under	over

Overall in Table 2, this meal is not too far off in terms of calories. This person wants to lose 20 pounds, and the range between maintenance and extreme weight loss is 1860 - 1360. The total calories of 1508.5 fall somewhere in the middle. But the goal was 1488, and let's say low carb and high protein. Let's try again.

Table 3	Carbs	Protein	Fat	Totals
Breakfast	Basted Egg with Smoked Salmon on Toast			
grams	28	13	19	
calories	112	52	171	335
Lunch	Citrus Pesto Chicken Salad			
grams	4	25	5	
calories	16	100	45	161
	Lemon Mustard Dressing			
grams	1	0	2	
calories	4	0	18	22
snack	Jumpin' Quinoa Munch Bars			
grams	12	2	4	
calories	48	8	36	92

	Carbs	Protein	Fat
GRAMS per day	93g	148g	57g
GRAMS per meal	18.6g	29.6g	11.4g
CALORIES per day	372 cals	595 cals	521 cals
CALORIES per meal	74.4 cals	119 cals	104.2 cals

Female, age: 55, weight: 170 lbs, height: 5' 4"

Goal: Lose 20 lbs at a moderate pace

Information from www.freedieting.com
Using the Daily Caloric Needs Calculator

Macro Ratio: 25% carbs, 40% prot, 35% fat

dinner	Baked Greek Salmon in a Pouch			
grams	9	40	28	
calories	36	160	252	448
	Savory Herb Roasted Potatoes			
grams	23	3	4	
calories	92	12	36	140
	Side Salad			
grams	3	1	0.5	
calories	12	4	4.5	20.5
	Red Wine Vinaigrette			
grams	0.5	0	3	
calories	2	0	27	29
snack	Power Snack			
grams	1	11	9	
calories	4	44	81	129
Total G	81.5	95	74.5	
Total C	326	380	670.5	1376.5

Calories to maintain current weight: 1860

Calories for fat loss: 1488

Calories for extreme fat loss: 1360

Grams per day	93g	148g	57g
	under	under	over

On this second try in Table 3 we have reduced fat by changing the evening snack from nuts and cheese, to nuts and an egg. Calories look great, but protein is still way under, and fat is still about 20 grams too high. Let's see if we can do better.

Table 4	Carbs	Protein	Fat	Totals
Breakfast	Savory Egg Cups with Goat Cheese			
grams	5	14	11	
calories	20	56	66	175
	Creamy Parfait with Berries			
grams	11	10	6	
calories	44	40	54	138
	Citrus Pesto Salad, as a snack			
grams	4	25	5	
calories	16	100	45	161
Lunch	Shrimp Salad			
grams	16	30	15	
calories	64	120	135	319
	Lemon Mustard Dressing			
grams	1	0	2	
calories	4	0	18	22
snack	Jumpin' Quinoa Munch Bars			
grams	12	2	4	
calories	48	8	36	92
dinner	Lime Grilled Pork Tenderloin			
grams	2	40	12	
calories	8	160	108	276

	Carbs	Protein	Fat
GRAMS per day	93g	148g	57g
GRAMS per meal	18.6g	29.6g	11.4g
CALORIES per day	372 cals	595 cals	521 cals
CALORIES per meal	74.4 cals	119 cals	104.2 cals

Female, age: 55, weight: 170 lbs, height: 5' 4"

Goal: Lose 20 lbs at a moderate pace

Information from www.freedieting.com
Using the Daily Caloric Needs Calculator

Macro Ratio: 25% carbs, 40% prot, 35% fat

Calories for fat loss: 1488
Calories for extreme fat loss: 1360

	Savory Herb Roasted Potatoes			
grams	23	3	4	
calories	92	12	36	140
	Side Salad			
grams	3	1	0.5	
calories	12	4	4.5	20.5
	Red Wine Vinaigrette			
grams	0.5	0	3	
calories	2	0	27	29
snack	Power Snack			
grams	1	11	9	
calories	4	44	81	129
Total G	78.5	136	71.5	
Total C	314	544	610.5	1501.5

Grams per day	93g	148g	57g
	under	under	over

So in Table 4, we increased protein by changing the breakfast to egg cups and added a yogurt parfait. We moved the chicken pesto salad down as a mid-morning snack and added a shrimp salad for lunch. We also swapped the baked salmon for pork tenderloin. So protein is looking better, but our calories jumped up. We are still in the weight loss zone, but let's see if we can do even better.

Table 5	Carbs	Protein	Fat	Totals
Breakfast	Savory Egg Cups with Goat Cheese			
grams	5	14	11	
calories	20	56	66	175
	Creamy Parfait with Berries			
grams	11	10	6	
calories	44	40	54	138
Snack	Power Drink - by True Athlete			
grams	4	20	2	
calories	16	80	18	114
Lunch	Shrimp Salad			
grams	16	30	15	
calories	64	120	135	319
	Lemon Mustard Dressing			
grams	1	0	2	
calories	4	0	18	22
snack	Jumpin' Quinoa Munch Bars			
grams	12	2	4	
calories	48	8	36	92
dinner	Lime Grilled Pork Tenderloin			

	Carbs	Protein	Fat
GRAMS per day	93g	148g	57g
GRAMS per meal	18.6g	29.6g	11.4g
CALORIES per day	372 cals	595 cals	521 cals
CALORIES per meal	74.4 cals	119 cals	104.2 cals

Female, age: 55, weight: 170 lbs, height: 5' 4"

Goal: Lose 20 lbs at a moderate pace

Information from www.freedieting.com
Using the Daily Caloric Needs Calculator

Macro Ratio: 25% carbs, 40% prot, 35% fat

Calories to maintain current weight: 1860
Calories for fat loss: 1488
Calories for extreme fat loss: 1360

grams	2	40	12	
calories	8	160	108	276
	Savory Herb Roasted Potatoes			
grams	23	3	4	
calories	92	12	36	140
	Side Salad			
grams	3	1	0.5	
calories	12	4	4.5	20.5
	Red Wine Vinaigrette			
grams	0.5	0	3	
calories	2	0	27	29
snack	Power Drink - by True Athlete			
grams	4	20	2	
calories	16	80	18	114
Total G	81.5	140	61.5	
Total C	326	560	520.5	1439.5

Grams per day	93g	148g	57g
	close	close	close

Table 5 has a much better balance. So what did we change? We changed the mid-morning and evening snacks for a power drink (Ensure, Whey Protein, etc.). These drinks are basically powdered milk (whey) and cocoa powder. There is also a multitude of excellent sports drink powders on the market, but they tend to have high-carb levels because they are meant for workout boost.

21-Day Meal Plan

Note: This is a guide based on a female, 50, doing some exercise, working a sedentary job, and would like to lose 20 lbs. You need to tailor the meals to fit your goals.

Week 1

1	Breakfast	Portion	gCarbs	gProt	gFat	cCarbs	cProt	cFat	Calories
Br	Feta, Quinoa, Egg Muffin	2 muffins	12	13	15	48	52	135	235
Sn	Creamy Parfait with Berries	1/2	11	10	6	44	40	54	138
Ln	Citrus Pesto Chicken Salad	1/6	4	25	5	16	100	45	161
Sn	Protein Drink	1	4	20	2	16	80	18	114
Dn	Spicy Pan-Seared Salmon	1/4	0	33	17	0	132	153	285
	Steamed Asparagus	1/4	3	2	1	12	8	9	29
	Orzo Salad	1/4	13	5	11	52	20	99	171
Sn	Good Fat Snack	1	3	13	23	12	52	207	271
	Totals		50	121	80	200	484	720	1404

2	Breakfast	Portion	gCarbs	gProt	gFat	cCarbs	cProt	cFat	Calories
Br	Basted Egg with Smoked Salmon on Toast	1	28	13	19	112	52	171	335
Sn	Protein Drink	1	4	20	2	16	80	18	114

			gCarbs	gProt	gFat		cCarbs	cProt	cFat	Calories
Ln	Feta, Quinoa, Egg Muffin	2 muffins	12	13	15		48	52	135	235
	Side Salad	1/4	3	1	0.5		12	4	4.5	20.5
Sn	Protein Drink	1	4	20	2		16	80	18	114
Dn	Citrus Pesto Chicken Salad	1/6	4	25	5		16	100	45	161
	Almond Ricotta Spread with Fruit	1/6	31	9	10		124	36	90	250
Sn	Vegan No-Bake Cookies	1 cookie	8	3	7		32	12	63	107
	Yogurt Cheese Cake	1/10	15	6	3		60	24	27	111
	Totals		94	104	61		376	416	545	1447.5

3	Breakfast	Portion	gCarbs	gProt	gFat		cCarbs	cProt	cFat	Calories
Br	Sunny Breakfast Salad	1/4	19	12	16		76	48	144	268
Sn	None									0
Ln	Shrimp Sandwich with Bleu Cheese Dressing	1/4	60	43	26		240	172	234	646
Sn	Protein Drink	1	4	20	2		16	80	18	114
Dn	Lime Grilled Pork Tenderloin	1/6	2	40	12		8	160	108	276
	Steamed Asparagus	1/4	3	2	1		12	8	9	29
	Side Salad	1/4	3	1	0.5		12	4	4.5	20.5
Sn	Yogurt Cheese Cake	1/10	15	6	3		60	24	27	111
	Totals		106	124	61		424	496	545	1464.5

4	Breakfast	Portion	gCarbs	gProt	gFat	cCarbs	cProt	cFat	Calories
Br	Savory Egg Cups with Goat Cheese	2 cups	5	14	11	20	56	99	175
Sn	Vegan No-Bake Cookies	1 cookie	8	3	7	32	12	63	107
Ln	Greek Salad	1/4	25	39	23	100	156	207	463
Sn	Evening Pick-Me-Up	1/4	6	12	21	24	48	189	261
Dn	Baked Greek Salmon in a Pouch	1/4	9	40	28	36	160	252	448
	Steamed Asparagus	1/4	3	2	1	12	8	9	29
	Side Salad	1/4	3	1	0.5	12	4	4.5	20.5
Sn	Yogurt Cheese Cake	1/10	15	6	3	60	24	27	111
	Totals		74	117	95	296	468	851	1614.5

5	Breakfast	Portion	gCarbs	gProt	gFat	cCarbs	cProt	cFat	Calories
Br	Berry Breakfast Quinoa	1/4	54	12	8	216	48	72	336
Sn	Almond Ricotta Spread with Fruit	1/6	31	9	10	124	36	90	250
Ln	Savory Egg Cups with Goat Cheese	2 cups	5	14	11	20	56	99	175
	Orzo Salad	1/4	13	5	11	52	20	99	171
Sn	Protein Drink	1	4	20	2	16	80	18	114
Dn	Broiled Snapper	1/4	0	45	6	0	180	54	234

	Kale	1/6	1	1	2	4	4	18	26
	Cuc & Dill Salad	1/4	4	2	9	16	8	81	105
Sn	Yogurt Cheese Cake	1/10	15	6	3	60	24	27	111
	Totals		127	114	62	508	456	558	1522

6	Breakfast	Portion	gCarbs	gProt	gFat	cCarbs	cProt	cFat	Calories
Br	Whole Wheat Pancakes with Greek Yogurt Topping	2 cakes	31	10	9	124	40	81	245
	Whole Wheat Pancakes with Greek Yogurt Topping	2 cakes	31	10	9	124	40	81	245
Sn	None, we had 4 cakes								
Ln	Creamy Chicken Salad with Basil Pesto	1/6	6	21	22	24	84	198	306
	Vegan No-Bake Cookies	1 cookie	8	3	7	32	12	63	107
Sn	Protein Drink	1	4	20	2	16	80	18	114
Dn	Greek Salad	1/4	25	39	23	100	156	207	463
Sn	Vegan No-Bake Cookies	1 cookie	8	3	7	32	12	63	107
	Totals		113	106	79	452	424	711	1587

7	Breakfast	Portion	gCarbs	gProt	gFat	cCarbs	cProt	cFat	Calories
Br	Berry Breakfast Quinoa	1/4	54	12	8	216	48	72	336

Sn	Protein Drink	1		4	20	2		16	80	18	114
Ln	Creamy Chicken Salad with Basil Pesto	1/6		6	21	22		24	84	198	306
	Vegan No-Bake Cookies	1 cookie		8	3	7		32	12	63	107
Sn	Protein Drink	1		4	20	2		16	80	18	114
Dn	Mediterranean Shrimp Fajitas	1/4		35	43	10		140	172	90	402
Sn	Power Snack	1		1	11	9		4	44	81	129
	Totals			112	130	60		448	520	540	1508

Week 2

1	Breakfast	Portion	gCarbs	gProt	gFat	cCarbs	cProt	cFat	Calories
Br	Savory Egg Cups with Goat Cheese	2 cups	5	14	11	20	56	99	175
Sn	Almond Ricotta Spread with Fruit	1/6	31	9	10	124	36	90	250
Ln	Creamy Chicken Salad with Basil Pesto	1/6	6	21	22	24	84	198	306
Sn	Vegan No-Bake Cookies	1 cookie	8	3	7	32	12	63	107
	Protein Drink	1	4	20	2	16	80	18	114
Dn	Rosemary & Spinach Frittata	1/8	5	10	10	20	40	90	150
	Side Salad	1/4	3	1	0.5	12	4	4.5	20.5
	Savory Herb Roasted Potatoes	1/4	23	3	4	92	12	36	140
Sn	Protein Drink	1	4	20	2	16	80	18	114
	Totals		89	101	69	356	404	617	1376.5

2	Breakfast	Portion	gCarbs	gProt	gFat	cCarbs	cProt	cFat	Calories
Br	Berry Breakfast Quinoa	1/4	54	12	8	216	48	72	336
Sn	Protein Drink	1	4	20	2	16	80	18	114
Ln	Arugula Shrimp Salad with White	1/4	23	34	9	92	136	81	309

	Beans								
Sn	Protein Drink	1	4	20	2	16	80	18	114
Dn	Baked Greek Salmon in a Pouch	1/4	9	40	28	36	160	252	448
	Steamed Asparagus	1/4	3	2	1	12	8	9	29
	Side Salad	1/4	3	1	0.5	12	4	4.5	20.5
Sn	Protein Drink	1	4	20	2	16	80	18	114
	Totals		104	149	53	416	596	473	1484.5

3	Breakfast	Portion	gCarbs	gProt	gFat	cCarbs	cProt	cFat	Calories
Br	Savory Egg Cups with Goat Cheese	2 cups	5	14	11	20	56	99	175
Sn	Citrus Pesto Chicken Salad	1/6	4	25	5	16	100	45	161
Ln	Dilled Chicken on Quinoa	1/4	18	30	23	72	120	207	399
Sn	Protein Drink	1	4	20	2	16	80	18	114
Dn	Mediterranean Shrimp Fajitas	1/4	35	43	10	140	172	90	402
	Beet Salad	1/6	7	2	9	28	8	81	117
	Side Salad	1/4	3	1	0.5	12	4	4.5	20.5
Sn	Jumpin' Quinoa Munch Bars	1 Bar	12	2	4	48	8	36	92
	Totals		88	137	65	352	548	581	1480.5

4	Breakfast	Portion	gCarbs	gProt	gFat	cCarbs	cProt	cFat	Calories
Br	Basted Egg with Smoked Salmon on Toast	1	28	13	19	112	52	171	335

Sn	Protein Drink	1	4	20	2	16	80	18	114
Ln	Citrus Pesto Chicken Salad	1/6	4	25	5	16	100	45	161
Sn	Protein Drink	1	4	20	2	16	80	18	114
Dn	Greek-Style Grouper	1/4	0	42	9	0	168	81	249
	Kale	1/6	1	1	2	4	4	18	26
	Side Salad	1/4	3	1	0.5	12	4	4.5	20.5
	Sun-Kissed Quinoa	1/6	22	7	7	88	28	63	179
Sn	Mediterranean Mousse	1/4	28	9	10	112	36	90	238
	Totals		94	138	57	376	552	509	1436.5

5	Breakfast	Portion	gCarbs	gProt	gFat	cCarbs	cProt	cFat	Calories
Br	Berry Breakfast Quinoa	1/4	54	12	8	216	48	72	336
Sn	Protein Drink	1	4	20	2	16	80	18	114
Ln	Savory Egg Cups with Goat Cheese	2 cups	5	14	11	20	56	99	175
	Side Salad	1/4	3	1	0.5	12	4	4.5	20.5
Sn	Protein Drink	1	4	20	2	16	80	18	114
Dn	Arugula Shrimp Salad with White Beans	1/4	23	34	9	92	136	81	309
	Mediterranean Mousse	1/4	28	9	10	112	36	90	238
Sn	Protein Drink	1	4	20	2	16	80	18	114
	Totals		125	130	45	500	520	401	1420.5

6	Breakfast	Portion	gCarbs	gProt	gFat	cCarbs	cProt	cFat	Calories

Br	Basted Egg with Smoked Salmon on Toast	1	28	13	19	112	52	171	335
Sn	Protein Drink	1	4	20	2	16	80	18	114
Ln	Shrimp Salad	1/4	16	30	15	64	120	135	319
Sn	Jumpin' Quinoa Munch Bars	1 Bar	12	2	4	48	8	36	92
Dn	Spicy Pan-Seared Salmon	1/4	0	33	17	0	132	153	285
	Steamed Asparagus	1/4	3	2	1	12	8	9	29
	Side Salad	1/4	3	1	0.5	12	4	4.5	20.5
Sn	Evening Pick-Me-Up	1/4	6	12	21	24	48	189	261
	Totals		72	113	80	288	452	716	1455.5

7	Breakfast	Portion	gCarbs	gProt	gFat	cCarbs	cProt	cFat	Calories
Br	Whole Wheat Pancakes with Greek Yogurt Topping	2 cakes	31	10	9	124	40	81	245
Sn	Protein Drink	1	4	20	2	16	80	18	114
Ln	Breakfast Casserole for Eight	1/8	36	15	15	144	60	135	339
Sn	none								
Dn	Baked Greek Salmon in a Pouch	1/4	9	40	28	36	160	252	448
	Kale	1/6	1	1	2	4	4	18	26
	Cuc & Dill Salad	1/4	4	2	9	16	8	81	105

Sn	Mediterranean Mousse	1/4	28	9	10		112	36	90	238
	Totals		113	97	75		452	388	675	1515

Week 3

1	Breakfast	Portion	gCarbs	gProt	gFat	cCarbs	cProt	cFat	Calories
Br	Feta, Quinoa, Egg Muffin	2 muffins	12	13	15	48	52	135	235
Sn	Creamy Parfait with Berries	1/2	11	10	6	44	40	54	138
Ln	Citrus Pesto Chicken Salad	1/6	4	25	5	16	100	45	161
Sn	Protein Drink	1	4	20	2	16	80	18	114
Dn	Greek Flank Steak	1/6	1	43	21	4	172	189	365
	Steamed Asparagus	1/4	3	2	1	12	8	9	29
	Orzo Salad	1/4	13	5	11	52	20	99	171
	Savory Herb Roasted Potatoes	1/4	23	3	4	92	12	36	140
Sn	Power Snack	1	1	11	9	4	44	81	129
	Totals		72	132	74	288	528	666	1482

2	Breakfast	Portion	gCarbs	gProt	gFat	cCarbs	cProt	cFat	Calories
Br	Almond Ricotta Spread with Fruit	1/6	31	9	10	124	36	90	250
Sn	Protein Drink	1	4	20	2	16	80	18	114
Ln	Greek Flank Steak	1/6	1	43	21	4	172	189	365
	Side Salad	1/4	3	1	0.5	12	4	4.5	20.5
Sn	Vegan No-Bake Cookies	1 cookie	8	3	7	32	12	63	107
Dn	Citrus Pesto Chicken Salad	1/6	4	25	5	16	100	45	161

		Portion	gCarbs	gProt	gFat	cCarbs	cProt	cFat	Calories
	Almond Ricotta Spread with Fruit	1/6	31	9	10	124	36	90	250
Sn	Vegan No-Bake Cookies	1 cookie	8	3	7	32	12	63	107
	Yogurt Cheese Cake	1/10	15	6	3	60	24	27	111
	Totals		90	113	63	360	452	563	1485.5

3	Breakfast	Portion	gCarbs	gProt	gFat	cCarbs	cProt	cFat	Calories
Br	Sunny Breakfast Salad	1/4	19	12	16	76	48	144	268
Sn	None								0
Ln	Shrimp Sandwich with Bleu Cheese Dressing	1/4	60	43	26	240	172	234	646
Sn	Protein Drink	1	4	20	2	16	80	18	114
Dn	Lime Grilled Pork Tenderloin	1/6	2	40	12	8	160	108	276
	Steamed Asparagus	1/4	3	2	1	12	8	9	29
	Side Salad	1/4	3	1	0.5	12	4	4.5	20.5
Sn	Yogurt Cheese Cake	1/10	15	6	3	60	24	27	111
	Totals		106	124	61	424	496	545	1464.5

4	Breakfast	Portion	gCarbs	gProt	gFat	cCarbs	cProt	cFat	Calories
Br	Basted Egg with Smoked Salmon on Toast	1	28	13	19	112	52	171	335

Sn	None								
Ln	Greek Salad	1/4	25	39	23		100	156	207	463
Sn	Jumpin' Quinoa Munch Bars	1 Bar	12	2	4		48	8	36	92
Dn	Spicy Pan-Seared Salmon	1/4	0	33	17		0	132	153	285
	Steamed Asparagus	1/4	3	2	1		12	8	9	29
	Side Salad	1/4	3	1	0.5		12	4	4.5	20.5
Sn	Yogurt Cheese Cake	1/10	15	6	3		60	24	27	111
	Totals		86	96	68		344	384	608	1335.5

5	Breakfast	Portion	gCarbs	gProt	gFat		cCarbs	cProt	cFat	Calories
Br	Berry Breakfast Quinoa	1/4	54	12	8		216	48	72	336
Sn	Jumpin' Quinoa Munch Bars	1 Bar	12	2	4		48	8	36	92
Ln	Savory Egg Cups with Goat Cheese	2 cups	5	14	11		20	56	99	175
	Orzo Salad	1/4	13	5	11		52	20	99	171
Sn	Protein Drink	1	4	20	2		16	80	18	114
Dn	Broiled Snapper	1/4	0	45	6		0	180	54	234
	Kale	1/6	1	1	2		4	4	18	26
	Cuc & Dill Salad	1/4	4	2	9		16	8	81	105
Sn	Yogurt Cheese Cake	1/10	15	6	3		60	24	27	111
	Totals		108	107	56		432	428	504	1364

6	Breakfast	Portion	gCarbs	gProt	gFat	cCarbs	cProt	cFat	Calories
Br	Whole Wheat Pancakes with Greek Yogurt Topping	2 cakes	31	10	9	124	40	81	245
	Whole Wheat Pancakes with Greek Yogurt Topping	2 cakes	31	10	9	124	40	81	245
Sn	None, we had 4 cakes								
Ln	Creamy Chicken Salad with Basil Pesto	1/6	6	21	22	24	84	198	306
	Vegan No-Bake Cookies	1 cookie	8	3	7	32	12	63	107
Sn	Protein Drink	1	4	20	2	16	80	18	114
Dn	Broiled Snapper	1/4	0	45	6	0	180	54	234
	Steamed Asparagus	1/4	3	2	1	12	8	9	29
	Side Salad	1/4	3	1	0.5	12	4	4.5	20.5
Sn	Vegan No-Bake Cookies	1 cookie	8	3	7	32	12	63	107
	Totals		94	115	64	376	460	572	1407.5

7	Breakfast	Portion	gCarbs	gProt	gFat	cCarbs	cProt	cFat	Calories
Br	Berry Breakfast Quinoa	1/4	54	12	8	216	48	72	336
Sn	Protein Drink	1	4	20	2	16	80	18	114
Ln	Citrus Pesto	1/6	4	25	5	16	100	45	161

	Chicken Salad								
	Vegan No-Bake Cookies	1 cookie	8	3	7	32	12	63	107
Sn	Protein Drink	1	4	20	2	16	80	18	114
Dn	Shrimp Salad	1/4	16	30	15	64	120	135	319
	Almond Ricotta Spread with Fruit	1/6	31	9	10	124	36	90	250
Sn	Power Snack	1	1	11	9	4	44	81	129
	Totals		122	130	58	488	520	522	1530

Chapter 4: Altering the Meal Plan to Fit Your Goals

Shredding: Weight Loss Goal

This is a term used to describe a rigid diet and workout schedule with the goal of burning fat and losing weight. This method relies heavily on cardiovascular exercises such as swimming, cycling, jogging, and treadmill and using equipment such as elliptical trainers.

Shed workouts also use weight training, but not with the goal of adding muscle. The goal is to keep the heart rate in the fat-burning zone by keeping the speed and intensity up.

Bulking: Build Muscle Mass

Bulking refers to building up big, bulky muscles. Think Arnold Schwarzenegger. Doing shorter reps with heavier weights is the goal. A diet high in protein is the key. After all, as we learned earlier, protein builds and repairs tissues in the body but is not stored in the body.

Special Diet: Questions for Your Physician

- What should my weight goal be?
- What macro ratio do I want to use for my goal?
- Let your physician know about any medicines you take.
- Tell him your exercise routine, or ask him to help you set up a routine.
- Some health plans have councilors to guide patients. See if your health care offers this option.
- If you don't have a health care plan, start walking. Walk around the block and see how you feel. Add on more minutes each week, until you feel comfortable with a 40-minute walk 4 or 5 times a week.

Chapter 5: Breakfast

1. Basted Egg With Smoked Salmon on Toast

~ This tastes as good as it looks and is quick and easy ~

Ingredients

- Whole grain toast (1 slice)
- Avocado (half)
- A squeeze of lemon or lime
- Salt and pepper (to taste)
- Microgreens (optional - to reduce carbs, serve on 1 c greens)
- Wild lox salmon (1 oz.)
- Egg, poached or basted (1 egg)
- Chopped green onions (optional)
- Dash of soy sauce (optional)

Tools

- Small saucepan (for 1 or 2 servings poached)
- Large, nonstick skillet with cover (for 3 to 6 servings basted)
- Small, stainless mixing bowl (1.5 qt.)
- Slotted spoon
- Fork
- Paring knife
- Toaster or broiler

Serves: 1

Per Serving: 28g, 13g, 19g = 112+52+171 = 335 calories

Directions:

1. This recipe is fast and easy, so you want to have all your ingredients out and ready to go.

2. Fill the small saucepan three-quarters full with water and place over high heat, with the lid on, and bring it to boil. Remove lid, and turn the heat down to a simmer.

3. While heating the water, pit and peel half an avocado. Place in a small mixing bowl. Squeeze in about a tablespoon of lemon or lime juice, and add a pinch of salt. Coarsely mash the avocado to mix in juice and salt. You want large bites of avocado, not a spreading consistency.

4. Stir in fast clockwise circles to create a small vortex at the center of the pan. Gently crack an egg into the center of the swirl. Get your egg as close as you can to the water before releasing from the shell. Allow cooking for 1-2 minutes until the yolk reaches the consistency you enjoy.

5. Chop the green onion.

6. Toast your bread.

7. While the bread is toasting, your egg should be ready. You want to remove it from the pan

with a slotted spoon and set the spoon on a folded paper towel to drain any water. Leave the egg resting in the spoon; don't try to blot the egg. If you see water on top of the egg, tilt slightly to drain.

8. Assembly time! Place your toast on a plate, and spread the avocado mixture on the toast. Arrange the smoked salmon on top of the avocado, with some microgreens on top of the salmon. Gently slide your poached egg to the center and top with a splash of soy sauce and chopped green onions.

9. Enjoy - I love this breakfast.

2. Breakfast Casserole for Eight

~ Great for a crowd, breakfast picnic, or brunch at the office ~

Ingredients

- Cooked quinoa (2 c)
- Sea salt and pepper (to taste)
- Fresh cilantro or parsley, chopped (2 T)
- Half & half cream (.3 c - use skim milk to reduce fat)
- Large eggs (8)
- Feta cheese, crumbled (3 oz.)
- Dried oregano (.5 tea)
- Fresh basil, gently torn or cut (1 T)
- Kalamata olives, chopped (.5 c)
- Fresh spinach leaves (5 oz.)
- Grape tomatoes, halved (1 c)
- Garlic, minced (2 cloves)
- Red bell pepper, finely diced (1 med)
- Yellow onion, finely diced (1 sm)
- Olive oil (2 T)
-

Tools

- 3 qt pan with lid
- 3 qt bowl
- 12" nonstick skillet
- Measuring cup (2 c)
- Measuring spoons
- Wisk
- Veggie knife, spatula, large mixing spoon

Serves: 8

Per Serving (1/8): 36g, 15g, 15g = 144 + 60 + 135 = 339 calories

Directions:

1. Lightly grease a 9 x 13 Pyrex pan, and set your oven to 350 degrees to pre-heat.

2. Bring to boil 1 cup of quinoa with 2 cups water, and reduce heat to simmer for 15 - 20 minutes until the liquid is almost absorbed. Take off heat, and let it sit to cool and finish absorbing liquid.

3. While quinoa is cooking, saute onions and garlic in olive oil over medium-high heat for 2-3 minutes until onions start to turn translucent; add in bell pepper after 2 minutes.

4. Stir in basil, oregano, cherry tomatoes, olives, and fresh spinach until spinach is wilted down.

5. Stir in quinoa and add salt and pepper to taste.

6. Spread quinoa mixture into the casserole pan evenly, and top with feta cheese.

7. Break eggs into a medium bowl, and whisk in cream or milk with salt and pepper to taste. Pour egg mixture over the casserole and top with cilantro or parsley.

8. Bake uncovered for 30 minutes or until the eggs are set. This may be served hot or cold, and it keeps in the refrigerator for up to five days.

3. Almond Ricotta Spread With Fruit

~ This is another yummy, quick start to the day ~

Ingredients

- Zest from orange, optional
- Honey (1 tea)
- Almond extract (.25 tea)
- Almonds (sliced) (.5 c)
- Whole milk ricotta (1 c)

Serving

- Whole grain bread, English muffing or bagel, toasted
- Peaches, sliced (.5 peach per serving)
- Extra almonds, sliced
- Extra honey (drizzle)

Tools

- Medium stainless mixing bowl
- Paring knife
- Mixing spoon
- Measuring spoons

Serves: 4-6

Per Serving (1/6): 31g, 9g, 10g = 124 + 36 + 90 = 250 calories

Directions:

1. Gently stir together orange zest, ricotta, almond extract, and almonds in a mixing bowl. Spoon into a serving bowl and top with additional sliced almonds and a drizzle of honey. This may be made ahead of time and stored in the refrigerator.

2. Assembly: Toast your bread. Spread a hearty tablespoon of ricotta on each piece of bread and top with sliced peaches, almonds, and a drizzle of honey.

4. Savory Egg Cups With Goat Cheese

~ It's a breakfast sandwich without all the carbs ~

Ingredients

- Roasted red bell peppers, chopped (1.5 c)
- Button mushrooms, chopped (1.5 c)
- Sea salt and fresh ground black pepper (to taste)
- Garlic, crushed and minced (small clove)
- Skim milk (.66 c)
- Eggs (10)
- Olive oil or cooking spray

Finishing

- Goat cheese, crumbled
- Fresh basil, torn

Tools

- Muffin tin (12 cups)
- Stainless bowl (large)
- Wisk
- Ladle
- Cooking spray

Serves: 6

Per Serving (2 cups): 5g, 14g, 11g = 20 + 56 + 99 = 175 calories

Directions:

1. Spray 12-cup muffin tin with cooking spray. Make sure to spray the top, as muffins can cook over. Set oven at 350 degrees.

2. Whisk eggs, milk, and minced garlic together in a large bowl. Season to taste. Add mushrooms and roasted red peppers, and stir thoroughly. Fill each muffin cup with the egg mixture; an ice cream scoop or ladle works well for this process. Use the entire mixture to fill all the cups.

3. When the oven is hot, bake for 25 minutes or until set.

4. Remove from oven, and let cool in the pan for 5-10 minutes, then turn from muffin tin. Use a knife to sweep around the side of each cup and pop the egg cups out.

5. Top with goat cheese and basil. These keep well in the refrigerator and can be packed as a to-go breakfast. Enjoy!

5. Sunny Breakfast Salad

~ Refreshing for a late breakfast on a warm summer day ~

Ingredients

- Quinoa, cooked and cooled (1 c)
- Eggs, soft-boiled (4)
  Note: Quinoa and eggs can be made the night before

- Arugula or spring mix (4 c)
- Grape tomatoes, halved (1 c)
- Cucumber, seeded and sliced (1 med)
- Hass avocado, sliced (2)
- Sea salt and fresh ground pepper (to taste)
- Lemon juice (2 T)
- Olive oil (4 tea)
- Fresh mint and dill, chopped (.5 c)
- Almonds, chopped (.5 c)

Tools

- Saucepans (medium, small)
- Measuring cups and spoons
- Paring knife
- Slotted spoon

Serves: 4

Per Serving (1/4): 19g, 12g, 16g = 76 + 48 + 144 = 268 calories

Directions:

1. If you don't have some quinoa already cooked, bring one cup of water to a boil, and add a pinch of salt and one-half cup of quinoa. Bring back to a boil, then turn the heat down to simmer (medium or lower). Let the quinoa simmer for 15 minutes. Stir, remove from heat, and let it finish absorbing the remaining water.

2. Soft-boil the eggs. In a small saucepan, bring water to a boil (enough to cover four eggs). Using a slotted spoon, gently lower eggs into the water and let simmer for 6 minutes.

3. Drain pan under cold running water, and gently tap each egg to dent the shell (makes them easier to peel later).

4. Combine quinoa, 1 tablespoon lemon juice, 2 teaspoons of olive oil, and salt, to taste.

5. In a large bowl, gently toss arugula, tomatoes, and herbs with 1 tablespoon lemon juice, 2 teaspoons of olive oil, and salt and pepper, to taste.

6. Peel your eggs.

7. Place arugula mixture on plates in four equal portions. Put a quarter of the quinoa mixture in the center of each plate. Arrange cucumber and avocado slices on the plate at opposite sides, and top salad with egg halves. Sprinkle almonds over the top. Add a pinch of seasoning to egg halves and a final drizzle of olive oil, and enjoy.

6. Berry Breakfast Quinoa

~ This hot, hearty breakfast will keep you going past noon ~

Ingredients

- Raw almonds, chopped (.25 c)
- Fresh berries (or your fresh fruit of choice) (.5 c)
- Honey (2 T) or substitute Stevia (2 tea to taste)
- Vanilla extract (1 tea)
- Sea salt (1 tea)
- Skim milk (2 c)
- Quinoa (1 c)
- Ground cinnamon (1 - 2 tea to taste)

Tools

- Two-quart saucepan
- Veggie knife
- Large spoon
- Measuring spoons

Serves: 4

Per Serving (1/4): 54g, 12g, 8g = 215.6 + 46 + 71.1 = 333 calories

Directions:

1. Toast nuts over medium heat 3-5 minutes until just brown. Stir or shake the pan every 40 seconds or so as nuts can easily burn. You can also use your microwave to toast nuts (try 30-sec increments until you find the right timing for your machine). Taste after every blast as items in the microwave burn from the inside out.

2. Add your quinoa grain and ground cinnamon to the saucepan, and heat the ingredients over medium heat until warm. Stir the milk and salt into the quinoa mixture over medium-high heat until mixture boils.

Lower heat to medium-low or low and simmer for 15 minutes. When the mixture has thickened and grain is tender, stir in vanilla, honey or stevia, fruit (reserve a few for topping), and about half of the almonds. Use the remaining nuts and fruit as toppings.

Note: If you are saving some or all for later in the week, do not add fruit. Wait until you reheat in the microwave before topping with fresh fruit as you go.

7. Caramelized Onion Egg Skillet

~ This recipe makes a great presentation. As pleasing to look at as it is to eat ~

Ingredients

- Whole grain toast, English muffin, Ciabatta rolls.
- Parsley, chopped (optional for topping)
- Sea salt and fresh ground pepper (to taste)
- Feta cheese, crumbled (3 oz)
- Large eggs (6-8)
- Julienne-cut sun-dried tomatoes, firmly packed (.3 c)
- Garlic, minced (1 clove)
- Olive oil (1T)
- Butter (1 T)
- Yellow onions, halved and sliced (4-5 small or 1.5 large)

Tools

- Large cast iron skillet with a lid (or use foil)
- Spatula

Serves: 6

Per Serving (1/6): 20g, 12g, 13g = 80 + 48 + 117 = 245 calories

Directions:

1. Heat olive oil and butter in a skillet over medium heat. When butter is melted and bubbly, add onion slices to the pan and coat with butter mixture. Spread onions across the pan in an even layer for a better result when browning. Lower heat to medium-low to low; onions should barely sizzle. Allow onions to cook for about 1 hour, stirring every 5-10 minutes until they are soft and deep brown.

2. When onions have the desired look, add garlic and sun-dried tomatoes. Stir gently, cooking for another 1-3 minutes until garlic is starting to soften.

3. Spread the mixture into an even layer, and carefully crack eggs over the top of the onion mixture. Season to taste and sprinkle feta cheese crumbles over the top. Cover tightly with lid or foil, and allow to cook for 10-15 minutes. Heat should still be on med-low to low. Watch the yolks in the last several minutes. Jiggle the pan to check doneness. Runny yolks will jiggle slightly. If you like your yolks well-done, they shouldn't move at all.

4. Remove from heat, and top with chopped parsley. Serve on crusty bread of your choice.

8. Rosemary & Spinach Frittata

~ This all-around favorite is great for parties ~

Ingredients

- Balsamic vinegar reduction (2 T)
- Eggs, beaten (8)
- Fresh lemon juice (2 tea)
- Fresh rosemary, minced (1 tea)
- Feta cheese, crumbled (3 oz or .75 c)
- Parmesan cheese, grated (1 oz or .3 c)
- Green onions, both white and green parts thinly sliced diagonally (2)
- Yellow or red roasted pepper, peeled and diced (1)
- Garlic, minced (4 small cloves)
- Sea salt and fresh ground pepper
- Fresh spinach, stemmed and washed (2 10 oz bags)
- Olive oil (1.5 tea)

Tools

- Cast iron skillet (large)
- Measuring cups and spoons
- Wisk
- Colander

Serves: 8-10

Per Serving (1/8): 5g, 10g, 10g = 20 + 40 + 90 = 150 calories

Directions:

1. Set oven to heat at 325 degrees

2. In a large, cast iron skillet, heat .5 tea of olive oil over high heat. Add half spinach, garlic, and a pinch of salt and pepper. When the leaves start to wilt (a minute or so), add the rest of the spinach and another pinch of salt and pepper. Drain and cool spinach in a colander over a stainless bowl to catch liquid).

3. Squeeze out extra liquid a handful at a time and transfer to cutting board for a rough chop.

4. In a large mixing bowl, whisk eggs together with a pinch of salt and pepper.

5. To the egg mixture, add and mix well the chopped spinach, lemon juice, feta, parmesan, green onions, and roasted pepper.

6. Over high heat, add remaining olive oil to saute pan, and heat almost to the smoking point, swirling the pan to coat sides with oil. Pour egg mixture into pan (eggs should sizzle), and reduce heat to low. Cook until sides begin to set, about 1-2 minutes. Transfer to oven and bake for 20-25 minutes or until eggs are golden and set.

7. Run a spatula around the rim to loosen sides of the frittata. Gently run a spatula under the frittata to help separate it from the bottom of the pan, as it can stick. Place a large plate upside down on top of the pan, then flip to turn the frittata out. Brush with balsamic reduction and serve.

9. Whole Wheat Pancakes With Greek Yogurt Topping

~ Indulge on a Sunday or a holiday ~

Ingredients

- Large egg (2)
- Buttermilk (2 c)
- Homemade pancake mix (2 c)

Topping

- Greek yogurt (1 c)
- Lemon, .25 zested (a pinch of zest)
- Almond extract (.25 tea or less)
- Blueberries, raspberries, blackberries, or mixed (1 c)

Tools

- Large nonstick skillet
- Spatula
- Large mixing bowl
- Wooden spoon
- Wisk
- Measuring cup

Serves: 8 (based on 16 pancakes)

Per Serving (2 cakes): 31g, 10g, 3g = 124 + 40 + 81 = 245 calories

Directions:

1. Whisk together 1 cup of mix, 1 cup of buttermilk (substitute .5 cup Greek yogurt and .5 cup skim milk if you do not have buttermilk), and egg in a large mixing bowl.

2. Let batter stand for 20 minutes for oats to soak up some of the liquid. The batter should thicken as it sits.

3. Heat skillet to medium-hot, and spoon batter into skillet to make 3" diameter cakes. About 1.5 spoonfuls make one cake, and you should be able to fit 3-4 cakes per pan.

4. After about 2 minutes, the edges of the cake should look dry, and bubbles should start to stay open and not fill back in with the batter. Turn cakes and finish cooking for about 2 more minutes. Stack first batch and repeat.

5. While pancakes are cooking, mix the first three topping ingredients.

6. Stack two or three cakes together and serve with a dollop of yogurt mixture topped with berries.

10. Homemade Whole Wheat Pancake Mix

Ingredients

- Safflower oil (1 c)
- Baking soda (1 T)
- Sea salt (1 T)
- Baking powder (3 T)
- Sugar (3 T or 1.5 T of stevia)
- Organic flour (1 c)
- Whole wheat flour (4 c)
- Old-fashioned rolled oats (3.5 c)

Tools

- Food processor
- Measuring cups and spoons

Yields: 10 cups or 50-80 pancakes

Per Cup (1/10): 73g, 10g, 24g = 292 + 40 + 216 = 548 calories

Directions:

1. Pulse oats in a food processor until finely ground; do not turn into a powder.

2. Using mixer fit with a paddle; add flours, oats, and all other dry ingredients. Mix slowly, adding safflower oil in a thin stream while the mixer is running.

3. Store in an airtight container in the refrigerator; it will keep good for months.

11. Feta, Quinoa, Egg Muffin

~ Pair these savory muffins with a bowl of fruit for a delicious start to the day ~

Ingredients

- Sea salt (.25 tea)
- Feta cheese, crumbled (1 c)
- Quinoa, cooked (1 c)
- Eggs (8)
- Safflower oil (2 tea)
- Cooking spray for muffin tins
- Dried oregano (1 tea)
- Kalamata olives, chopped (.5 c)
- Grape tomatoes, sliced (1 c)
- Yellow onion, finely chopped (1 small)
- Spinach, chopped (2 c)

Tools

- 12-cup muffin tin
- Veggie knife
- 12 nonstick skillet

Serves: 6

Per Serving (2 muffins): 12g, 13g, 15g = 48 + 52 + 135 = 235 calories

Directions:

1. Spray 12 cup muffin tin with cooking spray. Make sure to spray top, as muffins can cook over. Set oven at 350 degrees.

2. Add safflower oil and onions in the skillet under medium heat. Saute for 2 minutes, then add tomatoes and saute for another minute. Stir onion and tomato mixture; add spinach on top and allow to wilt (1 minute or so). Remove from the heat and mix in oregano and olives, then set aside.

3. In a large mixing bowl, whisk eggs until well-combined. Add cooled onion mixture, quinoa, and feta cheese to the egg mixture. Season to taste and mix well.

4. Using ladle or ice cream scoop, fill greased muffin tins with equal portions of the egg mixture. Bake for 30 minutes or until eggs have set and are light golden-brown on top. Cool for 5 minutes before serving. It may be eaten hot or cold or reheated in the microwave. It's great as a to-go breakfast.

12. Balsamic Vinegar Reduction

~ A touch of sweetness ~

This sweet and tart syrup is a wonderful addition to roasted vegetables, brushed-over baked egg dishes, or salads where it can be used with olive oil as dressing.

Ingredients

Basic balsamic vinegar (not the high-end variety that has already been reduced)

Directions:

1. Start with 1 cup balsamic vinegar in a small saucepan over high heat. Stirring occasionally, let vinegar boil until liquid thickens and has reduced in volume by about half.

2. Take it off the heat and allow to cool before storing in the refrigerator.

Chapter 6: Lunch Break

1. Shrimp Salad

~ Simple yet elegant ~

Ingredients
- Shrimp, cooked, deveined (1 lb large)
- Sliced beets, red or yellow (.5 c. from can)
- Orange slices (1 c.)
- Avocado slices (1 Hass)
- Gorgonzola crumbles (4 T)
- Mixed greens, packed (4 c.)
- Balsamic vinaigrette dressing (recipe to follow)

Tools
- Large pot with lid (3 qt)
- Colander
- Deveiner
- Paring knife
- Cutting board

Serves: 4
Per Serving (1/4): 16g, 30g, 15g = 64 + 120 + 135 = 319 calories

Directions:

1. You can cook the heads of the shrimp or clean them prior to cooking. If you choose to pull the heads off and devein prior to cooking, add the heads in the pot to get more flavor.

2. Let the water come to a boil in a large pot (at least two inches of water over the shrimp). Add a pinch of salt. You don't want to overcook the shrimp. A few will start to pop to the top when they are done. With larger shrimp, it may be 5-7 minutes. You want the shrimp to turn from

translucent to opaque at the thickest point.

3. Drain shrimp in colander; rinse in cold water and let cool.

4. Slice orange in half at the midsection. Cut around each wedge at the membrane, and pop out orange meat into a bowl. Do this for each half of the orange. You can squeeze the excess orange juice over the cooling, cleaned shrimp if you like.

5. If you did not clean shrimp before cooking, pull the heads and shell and devein now.

6. Assemble salads on the plates. Put equal portions of mixed greens on each plate. Arrange beets (4-5 slices) around the outer edge with avocado slices in between. Place shrimp (5-6) around the middle with orange wedges in between. Sprinkle the gorgonzola crumbs, and dress it lightly with balsamic vinaigrette.

2. Tropical Salad: Fruits, Nuts, & More

~ A tasty twist on the Spinach Salad ~

Ingredients

- Salad greens (1 c)
- Fresh spinach leaves (1 c)
- Apple, chopped (1)
- Lemon, half
- Walnuts, toasted and chopped (.5 c)
- Oranges, sliced (2)
- Sunflower Seeds (.5 c)
- Eggs, hard-boiled, peeled (4)
- Bacon, cooked slowly to render fat (4 slices)
- Gorgonzola cheese, crumbled

Tools

- Cast iron skillet (large)
- Meat fork
- Paring knife
- Measuring cup
- Small bowls (2)

Serves: 4

Per Serving (1/4): 23g, 21g, 28g = 92 + 84 + 252 = 428 calories

Directions:

1. Heat a skillet on medium-high heat, and add bacon strips. Turn heat down to medium or medium-low, and cook the bacon slowly to render out as much fat as possible. This takes 5-10 minutes, and you need to turn the bacon every 2 minutes or until the fat is golden brown. Remove from the pan and drain on paper towels.

2. Greens and spinach should be washed, drained, patted dry, stemmed, and chopped (if needed). Put equal portions on each of the four serving plates.

2. Toast walnuts in the microwave for at least 1.5 minutes (on paper towel).

3. Slice orange in half at center, not end to end. Run a knife around each wedge membrane, and pop out orange flesh into a small bowl. Repeat around the first half and continue with the second half.

4. Slice apple in two. With one half, slice lengthwise and then across widthwise to create small wedges. Do the same to the other half, and place them in a small bowl. Squeeze lemon juice over the apple wedges to keep them from turning brown while you are working.

5. Slice each egg and spread over greens as you move from plate to plate. Distribute equal portions of apples, oranges, sunflower seeds, and walnuts.

6. Crumble one piece of bacon over each plate. Finish with gorgonzola crumbles and serve with a carafe of Poppy Seed Dressing.

3. Greek Salad

~ *A Tampa favorite* ~

Ingredients
- Shrimp, cooked and deveined (1 lb large)
- Beets, sliced (1 can)
- Red onion, sliced into thin rings
- Olives, Kalamata and green (8 each)
- Eggs, hard boiled (4)
- Green pepper, sliced into rings (1 large)
- Feta cheese crumbles (.5 cup)
- Potato Salad (2 c)
- Mixed greens (4 c)
- Lemon Dressing

Tools
- Large pot with lid (3 qt)
- Shrimp deveiner
- Paring knife

Serves: 4
Per Serving (1/4): 25g, 39g, 23g = 100 + 156 + 207 = 463 calories

Directions:

1. You can cook the heads of the shrimp or clean them before cooking. If you choose to pull the heads off and devein prior to cooking, add the heads in the pot to get more flavor.

2. Let the water come to a boil in a large pot (at least two inches of water over the shrimp). Add a pinch of salt. Don't overcook the shrimp; a few will start to pop to the top when they are done. With larger shrimp, cooking may be 5-7 minutes. You want the shrimp to turn from translucent to opaque at the thickest point.

3. Drain shrimp in colander; rinse in cold water and let cool. If you did not clean shrimp prior to cooking, pull the heads and shell and devein now.

4. Assemble salads:

- Place a 1 cup of mixed greens on each of four plates.
- Place a scoop (.5 c) of potato salad in the center of the plate.
- Space beets (4-5), shrimp (5-6), and olives (2 Greek, 2 green) on greens, circling the potato salad.
- Quarter the eggs, and add to plate at four "corners."
- Arrange green pepper and onion rings across the top (2 or 3 of each).
- Sprinkle feta cheese over top and drizzle with lemon dressing. Enjoy!

4. Garbanzo Lettuce Wraps

~ Excellent choice for a high-energy day ~

Ingredients

- Green onions, sliced thin (.5 c)
- Roasted red peppers, drained and sliced (.5 c)
- Chickpeas, rinsed (2 (15 oz) cans)
- Tahini Lemon Dressing

Toppings

- Fresh parsley, chopped (2 T)
- Toasted almonds, chopped (.25 c)
- Bibb lettuce leaves (12 large)

Tools

- Can opener
- Paring knife
- Measuring cups and spoons
- Stainless bowl (large)

Serves: 4

Per Serving (1/4): 58g, 14g, 6g = 232 + 56 + 54 = 342 calories

Directions:

1. In a large bowl, add chickpeas, roasted red peppers, and green onions. Coat with Tahini Lemon Dressing and toss.

2. Spoon mixture into lettuce leaves, about a third cup each. Top with parsley and almonds. Roll leaves and serve, 3 to a plate.

5. Shrimp Sandwich With Bleu Cheese Dressing

~ Hot and delicious—an uptown Po Boy ~

Ingredients

- Shrimp, cooked and deveined (1 lb large)
- Herbed veggie spread (1 c)
- Bleu Cheese Dressing (.5 c)
- Mixed greens (1 cup)
- Plum tomatoes, sliced (2-3)
- Whole grain sub roll (4)

Tools
- Large pot with lid (3qt)
- Deveiner
- Baking sheet

Serves: 4
Per Serving (1/4): 60g, 43g, 26g = 240 + 172 + 234 = 646 calories

Directions:

1. You can cook the heads of the shrimp or clean them prior to cooking. If you choose to pull the heads off and devein before cooking, add the heads in the pot to get more flavor.

2. Let the water come to a boil in a large pot (at least two inches of water over shrimp). Add a pinch of salt. Do not overcook the shrimp; a few will start to pop to the top when they are done. With larger shrimp, cooking may be 5-7 minutes. You want the shrimp to turn from translucent to opaque at the thickest point.

3. Drain shrimp in colander; rinse in cold water and let cool. If you did not clean shrimp before cooking, pull heads and shell and devein now.

4. Arrange oven rack 4-6 inches from the heat source; set the oven to broil in high heat.

5. On a baking sheet, lay the four subs open-face. Spread herb Cheese on one side of the bun and layer with shrimp. Spread Bleu Cheese Dressing on the other half of bun and layer with tomatoes slices.

6. Put the baking sheet under the broiler for 30-60 seconds or until the edges of bun begin to toast.

7. Remove from oven and finish subs with a layer of lettuce and a drizzle of the Bleu Cheese Dressing.

6. Citrus Pesto Chicken Salad

~ *Chicken Salad with a twist* ~

Ingredients
- Chicken breast, boiled, chopped or shredded (4 6-oz)
- Celery, diced (1.5 c)
- Red bell pepper, diced (.75 c)
- Yellow squash, cored and sliced (.5 c)
- Citrus Pesto (1.5 T)
- Plain Greek yogurt (2 T)
- Olive oil (.5 tea)
- Sea salt and fresh ground pepper (to taste)
- Mixed greens (3 c)
- Parsley, roughly chopped for garnish
- Kalamata olives (12)
- Paprika

Tools
- Veggie knife
- Paring knife
- Stainless bowl (medium)

Serves: 6 salads
Per Serving (1/6): 4g, 25g, 5g = 16 + 100 + 45 = 161 calories

Directions:
1. Combine chicken breast, Citrus Pesto, yogurt, olive oil, salt, and pepper.
2. Add to this mixture: squash, bell pepper, and celery and fold in gently.
3. Divide greens equally over salad plates and top with equal parts chicken salad. Garnish with a sprinkle of paprika, parsley leaves, and a few Greek olives.
4. Serve with Lemon-Mustard Dressing and toasted pita wedges.

7. Pan Bagna

~ A French classic—Salad Nicoise to-go ~

Ingredients
- Capers, drained (2 T)
- Green onion, trimmed and minced (1 bunch)
- Kalamata olives, pitted and coarsely chopped (.5 c)
- Green beans, cleaned, stemmed, and blanched (2 c)
- Lemon zest (2 tea)
- Fresh basil, shredded (.25 c)
- Fresh lemon juice (.3 c)
- Garlic, minced (2 cloves)
- Olive oil (.5 c)
- Sea salt and fresh ground pepper (to taste)
- Vine-ripened tomatoes, sliced (2-3)
- Roasted red bell peppers, diced (.5 c)
- Mixed greens
- Tuna Salad (2 c)
- Whole grain baguette (2 15"-loaves). Cut in thirds for 6 5" subs

Tools
- Saucepan (3 qt)
- Colander
- Veggie knife
- Zester
- Ziploc bag or some airtight container (1 gal)
- Stainless bowl (large)

Serves: 6 subs
Per Serving (1/6): 52g, 20g, 20g = 208 + 80 + 180 = 468 calories

Directions:

1. Bring water in saucepan to a boil, add a pinch of sea salt, and gently drop in your green beans. The beans have previously been washed, drained, and stemmed, and the strings have been removed (pop off the stem and pull down; the string should come with the stem). Let the beans sit in water on the stove for 3 minutes.

2. Remove from heat and drain in a colander, running beans under cold water to stop the cooking process. This is called blanching. You are heating the outside of the vegetable just long enough to set the color, keep more nutrients in, and kill bacteria on the outside.

3. In a bowl, combine and toss capers, green onions, cooled green beans (yes, they are still whole), olives, lemon zest, roasted red pepper, and basil. In a smaller bowl, whisk together the lemon juice and garlic. Slowly whisk in the oil to make a vinaigrette. Season with salt and pepper and pour over the green bean mixture, tossing well.

4. Split the baguettes in half horizontally, and cut them into three sections of 5 inches each. Divide the Tuna Salad between the 6 rolls, spreading on one half of each roll, about .3 cup per roll.

5. Top tuna with sliced tomatoes and mixed greens. Top the other half of the sandwich with the green bean mixture and spoon some extra marinade on the roll. Sandwich the halves back together and let stand for at least 1 hour to let the dressing seep into the bread. Serve with plenty of napkins.

8. Tuna Salad

~ This works great as a high-protein, low-fat snack ~

Ingredients
- Tuna, white albacore in olive oil (5 oz can)
- Wickles Relish (1 T)
- Yellow mustard (1 tea)
- Sea salt and fresh ground pepper (to taste)
- Celery, diced (2 stalks)
- Green onions, diced, use green and white (1 stalk)
- Dash of cider vinegar (.5 tea)
- Eggs, hard boiled (2) — Omit eggs if you are using this for Pan Bagna

Tools
- Veggie knife
- Cutting board
- Measuring spoons
- Stainless bowl (small)

Serves: 4
Per Serving (1/4): 2g, 12g, 5g = 8 + 48 + 45 = 101 calories

Directions:

1. Drain tuna, place in a small bowl (I give the oil to my cats), and fork apart to make mixing easier. If you are making this for the Pan Bagna subs, skip to next step. Otherwise, chop eggs and mix into tuna.
2. Stir in relish, mustard, salt, pepper, and a dash of vinegar and mix well. To this mixture, add celery and green onions.

Eat with pita pockets or whole grain bread. I like to moisten the bread with butter then spread on tuna mixture. Top with lettuce and tomato, and enjoy.

9. Dilled Chicken on Quinoa

~ All components of this dish can be made ahead of time then assembled before serving or packing for a to-go lunch ~

Ingredients

- Fresh parsley, chopped (2 T)
- Feta cheese, crumbled (.25 c)
- Cucumber, sliced (1 c)
- Red onion, chopped fine (.25 c)
- Kalamata olives, chopped (.25 c)
- Quinoa, cooked (1 c)
- Crushed red pepper (.25 tea - optional)
- Ground cumin (.5 tea)
- Paprika (1 tea)
- Garlic, crushed (1 small clove)
- Olive oil (4 T)
- Almonds, slivered (.25 c)
- Roasted red peppers, rinsed (1, 7-oz jar)
- Dill weed (4 tea)
- Fresh ground pepper (.25 tea)
- Sea salt (.25)
- Chicken breast, boneless/skinless/trimmed (1 pound)

Tools

- Baking sheet
- Cooking spray
- Food processor

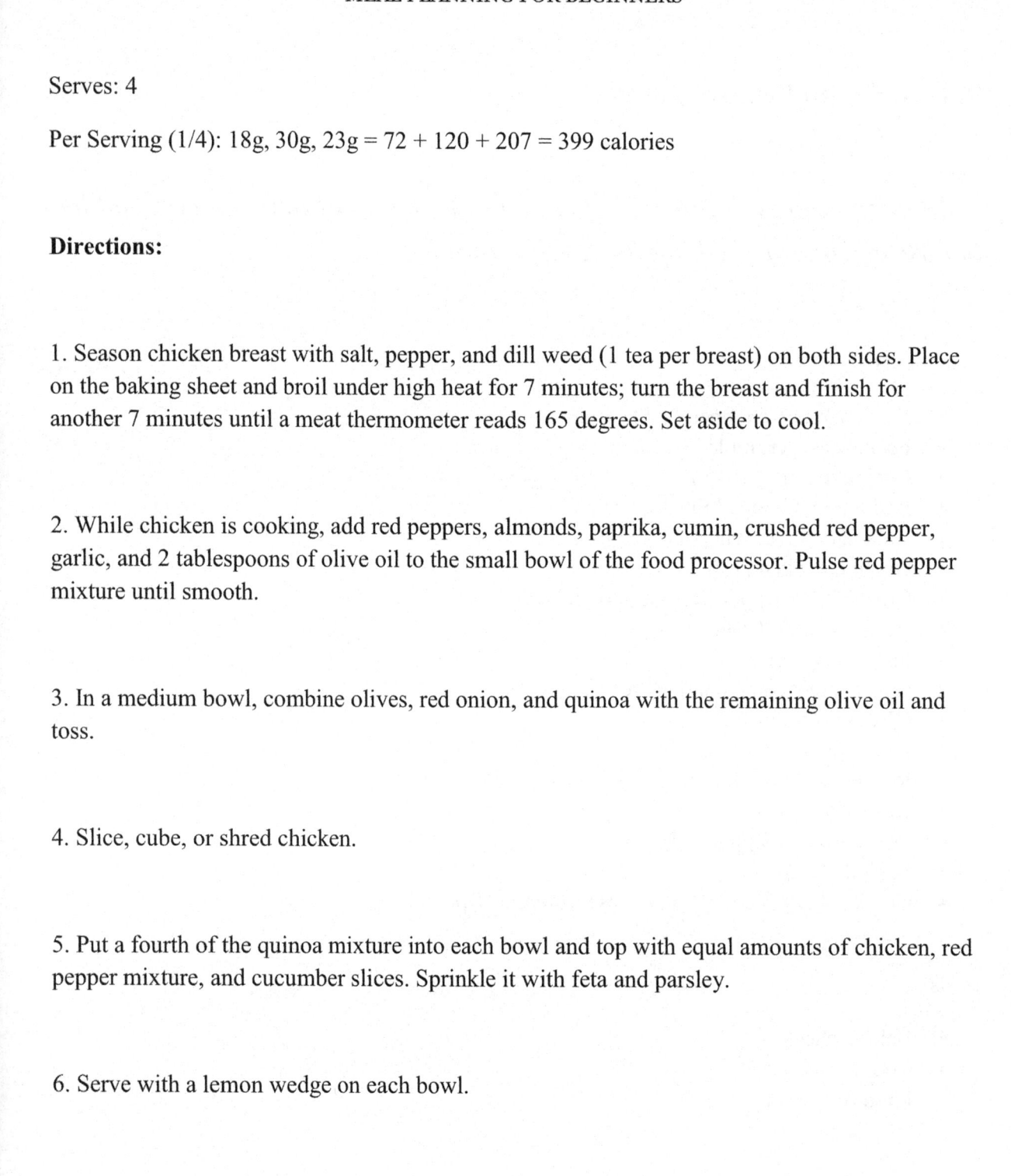

Serves: 4

Per Serving (1/4): 18g, 30g, 23g = 72 + 120 + 207 = 399 calories

Directions:

1. Season chicken breast with salt, pepper, and dill weed (1 tea per breast) on both sides. Place on the baking sheet and broil under high heat for 7 minutes; turn the breast and finish for another 7 minutes until a meat thermometer reads 165 degrees. Set aside to cool.

2. While chicken is cooking, add red peppers, almonds, paprika, cumin, crushed red pepper, garlic, and 2 tablespoons of olive oil to the small bowl of the food processor. Pulse red pepper mixture until smooth.

3. In a medium bowl, combine olives, red onion, and quinoa with the remaining olive oil and toss.

4. Slice, cube, or shred chicken.

5. Put a fourth of the quinoa mixture into each bowl and top with equal amounts of chicken, red pepper mixture, and cucumber slices. Sprinkle it with feta and parsley.

6. Serve with a lemon wedge on each bowl.

10. Creamy Chicken Salad With Basil Pesto

~ Makes a wonderful appetizer served on crackers ~

Ingredients

- Grape tomatoes, halved (.5 c)
- Arugula, chopped (1 c packed)
- Cooked chicken, shredded or chopped (3 c)
- Sea salt and fresh ground pepper (to taste)
- Lemon juice (2 tea)
- Pesto (2 T)
- Green onions, diced (2 T)
- Mayonnaise (.3 c)
- Greek yogurt (.5 c)

Toppings

- Toasted pine nuts (3 T - substitute walnuts or almonds)

Tools

- Stainless bowl (large)
- Paring knife
- Measuring cups

Serves: 6

Per Serving (1/6): 6g, 21g, 22g = 24 + 84 + 198 = 306 calories

Directions:

1. In a large bowl, add lemon juice, salt, pepper, pesto, and green onions and toss. To this, add mayonnaise and yogurt and stir. Fold in chicken and tomatoes.

2. Divide arugula evenly over the six serving plates. Top with an equal amount of chicken salad. Sprinkle on nuts and serve immediately or refrigerate for later.

11. Picnic Plate

~ *Mix and match—you get the idea* ~

Ingredients

- Whole wheat pita bread (4 4-inch)
- Vegan N0-Bake Cookies
- Pistachios, dry-roasted (.6 c)
- Blackberries, raspberries (1 c each). Can use sliced orange, fresh figs, or dried fruits if out of season.
- Mixed olives (1 c)
- Radishes (4)
- Sugar snap peas, stemmed (1 c)
- Beet Hummus (1 c)
- Tabbouleh (2 c)

Tools

- Colander to rinse fruit and veggies

Serves: 4

Per Serving (1/4): 57g, 14g, 15g = 228 + 56 + 135 = 419* calories

* Does not include cookie

Directions:

If packing for a picnic, place equal amounts in sealable containers. Pack pistachios, cookies, and pita separately, so they don't get soggy.

This is also a great work lunch choice.

12. Beet Hummus

~ A sweet change to an old favorite ~

Ingredients

- Sea salt (.5 tea)
- Ground cumin (1 tea)
- Garlic (1 clove)
- Lemon juice (.25 c)
- Olive oil (.25 c)
- Tahini (.25 c)
- Roasted beets or canned, chopped and patted dry (8 oz)
- Garbanzo beans, rinsed (1 15-oz can)

Tools

- Food processor
- Paring knife
- Lemon juicer
- Measuring cup and spoons
- Can opener

Serves: 10 (.25 c)

Per Serving (1/10): 29g, 10g, 6g = 116 + 40 + 54 = 210 calories

Directions:

Combine all ingredients in a food processor and pulse for 2-3 minutes until very smooth.

13. Hummus

~ You can snack, side, and salad all week! ~

Ingredients

- Sea salt (to taste)
- Ground cumin (1.5 T)
- Canned chickpeas, drained (6 c)
- Water (1 c)
- Tahini paste (1 c)
- Lemon juice (.5 c)
- Garlic, minced (3 large cloves)

Tools

- Food processor
- Stainless bowl (small)

Yield: 3.5 cups

Per Serving (.25 cup): 27g, 8g, 10g = 108 + 32 + 90 = 230 calories

Directions:

1. Combine tahini, lemon juice, and garlic in food processor and pulse until mixed. Add water, cumin, salt, and chickpeas. Process until mixture is smooth and creamy.

2. Place in a serving bowl and top with a sprinkle of paprika and a drizzle of olive oil. Garnish with lemon slices, Greek olives, and sprigs of fresh mint or parsley.

Note: For dips, use about a cup of hummus, sprinkle some paprika on top with a drizzle of olive oil, and serve with thick slices of cucumber, pita chips, carrot, and celery sticks.

14. Tabbouleh

~ Fresh ... crisp ... minty ~

Ingredients

- Fresh ground pepper (to taste)
- Parsley, flat leaf or curly, finely chopped (2 c)
- Tomatoes, diced (2)
- Fresh mint, chopped (.25 c)
- Sea salt (.25 tea)
- Garlic, minced (.5 tea)
- Olive oil (2 T)
- Lemon juice (.25 c)
- Bulgur wheat (.5 c)
- Water (1 c)
- Green onions, thinly sliced (4)
- Cucumber, peeled, seeded, and diced (1 small)

Tools

- Saucepan (medium)
- Stainless bowls (large, small)
- Measuring cups and spoons
- Veggie knife
- Cutting board

Serves: 4

Per Serving (1/4): 20g, 4g, 8g = 80 + 16 + 72 = 168 calories

Directions:

1. In a saucepan, add water and bulgur wheat and bring to a rolling boil. Remove from heat and let stand for 25 minutes or until bulgur wheat is tender. Transfer to a large mixing bowl.

2. In a small bowl, combine olive oil, lemon juice, garlic, salt, and pepper and whisk together. To bulgur wheat, add parsley, mint, cucumbers, tomatoes, and scallions. Dress with the lemon juice mixture and mix well. Serve at room temperature or chill for an hour to serve cold.

3. If you want to make it ahead and serve up to 4 days later, do not prepare cucumbers or tomatoes until you are ready to use and mix them in.

15. Balsamic Vinaigrette

~ *Herbal sweetness* ~

Ingredients
- Balsamic vinegar (1 c)
- Sugar (dash)
- Oregano (.5 tea)
- Thyme (.25)
- Fresh parsley, chopped fine (1 T)
- Sea salt (.5 tea)
- Fresh ground pepper (.5 tea)
- Garlic, minced (2 cloves)
- Olive oil (.25 c)

Tools
- Stainless bowl (medium)
- Wisk
- Paring knife
- Salad dressing carafe

Yields: 1.25 cup
Per Serving (1 T): 0.2g, 0g, 3g = .8 + 0 + 27 = 27.8 calories

Directions:

Combine vinegar, sugar, oregano, thyme, salt, pepper, and garlic. Whisk in olive oil (thin stream method). Stir in parsley and transfer to the carafe. Keep refrigerated until use.

16. Basic Pine Nut Pesto

~ Everybody's favorite ~

Ingredients

- Parmesan cheese, freshly grated (.5 c)
- Olive oil (.5 c)
- Garlic (2 cloves)
- Pine nuts (2 T) – you may use walnuts or pecans; have fun with variations
- Fresh basil leaves, stemmed (2 c)
  You can also play with the type of basil you use. Sweet basil is what cooks use the most. There are dark opal basil, lemon basil, Thai basil, holy basil (makes great tea), and more.

Tools

- Food processor
- Stainless bowl
- Rubber spatula
- Measuring cups

Yields: 1.25 cup

Per Serving (1 tablespoon): 0g, 1g, 6g = 0 + 4 + 54 = 58 calories

Directions:

1. Process (pulse, so you don't create mush) basil leaves, nuts, and garlic in a food processor until finely minced. With the machine on low, add oil in a thin stream until all oil is gone and the mixture is smooth. Stop processing; add the cheese and pulse to combine parmesan with basil mixture.

2. Refrigerate in an airtight container or freeze in Ziploc bag. Freezing works great. Spread the pesto out flat in the bag (about a quarter of an inch thick) and freeze flat. This way, when you are cooking, you can break off a bit and toss it in your dish without having to stop and make some. It can keep months in the freezer.

17. Lemon Tahini Dressing

~ Mouth watering ~

Ingredients

- Paprika (.25 tea)
- Sea salt (.5 tea)
- Honey (1.5 tea)
- Juice of two lemons (.25 c)
- Lemon zest (1 tea)
- Olive oil (.25 c)
- Tahini (.25 c)

Tools

- Stainless bowl (small)
- Wisk
- Dressing carafe

Yields: .75 cup

Per Serving (1 tablespoon): 2g, 1g, 7g = 8 + 4 + 63 = 75

Directions:

1. Whisk together all ingredients, and store it in the refrigerator until ready to use.

18. Lemon-Mustard Dressing

~ Tangy; goes great with almost everything ~

Ingredients
- Lemon juice (1 c)
- Cider vinegar (.5 c)
- Sugar (1 T)
- Oregano (.5 tea)
- Sea salt (.5 tea)
- Fresh ground pepper (.5 tea)
- Water (.25 c)
- Spicy brown mustard (1 T)
- Garlic, minced (2 cloves)
- Olive oil (.25 c)

Tools
- Stainless bowl (medium)
- Wisk
- Paring knife
- Salad dressing carafe or cruet

Yields: 2 cup
Per Serving (1 tablespoon): 1g, 0g, 2g = 4 + 0 + 18 = 22 calories

Directions:

Combine and mix well lemon juice, vinegar, sugar, oregano, salt, pepper, water, garlic, and mustard. Whisk in olive oil (thin stream method) and transfer to the carafe. Keep refrigerated until use.

19. Bleu Cheese Dressing

~ Should satisfy the fussiest bleu cheese lover ~

Ingredients
- Sugar (1-2 tea - to taste)
- Sea salt and fresh ground pepper (.5 tea each)
- Lemon juice (3 T)
- Cider vinegar (2 T)
- Bleu cheese, crumbled (1 c)
- Safflower oil (.66 c)
- Skim milk (.66 c)

Tools
- Food processor
- Zester
- Measuring spoons
- Measuring cup
- Salad dressing cruet

Yield: 2 cups
Per Serving (1 tablespoon): 1g, 1g, 6g = 4 + 4 + 54 = 62 calories

Directions:

1. Place bleu cheese and safflower oil in a food processor and pulse a few times until mixed.

2. Add in sugar, salt, pepper, cider vinegar, and lemon juice. Blend processor while adding the milk in a thin stream. Transfer dressing to salad dressing cruet and refrigerate.

20. Citrus Pesto

~ Try as a rub-on grilled chicken ~

Ingredients
- Lemon zest (.25 tea)
- Orange zest (.25 tea)
- Garlic, crushed (1 large clove)
- Sea salt and fresh ground pepper (to taste)
- Onion minced (.25 c)
- Parsley, chopped (2 c)
- Red pepper, cayenne (pinch)
- Green bell pepper, chopped (2 T)

Tools
- Zester
- Paring knife
- Stainless bowl (small)
- Measuring cups and spoons
- Chopping board

Yield: .5 cup
Per Serving (1 tablespoon): 4g, 1g, 0g = 16 + 4 + 0 = 20 calories

Directions:

Blend all ingredients together in a food processor to a smooth consistency. Store in refrigerator in an airtight container until ready to use.

21. Herb Veggie Spread

~ *A great substitute for mayonnaise* ~

Ingredients

- Yogurt Cheese (2 lb)
- Olive oil (.25 c)
- Sea salt (.5 tea - to taste)
- Sugar, stevia, or honey (2 tea - sugars, 1 tea stevia)
- Oregano (2 tea)
- Green and red bell pepper, chopped fine (1 each, medium)
- Carrots, peeled and grated (2 medium)

Tools

- Stainless bowl (medium)
- Measuring cups and spoons
- Veggie knife
- Veggie peeler

Yields: 4 cups

Per Serving (1/4 cup): 9g, 6g, 5g = 36 + 24 + 45 = 105 calories

Directions:

1. Combine yogurt cheese, olive oil, salt, and sugar in a bowl. Mix well.

2. Stir in bell peppers and grated carrots. Taste and adjust seasoning to taste. If you find the mixture bitter, add a small amount of sweetener at a time until you get the taste you desire.

22. Yogurt Cheese

~ A versatile ingredient similar to ricotta ~

Ingredients

- Non-homogenized plain yogurt (48 oz)

Tools

- Colander (large)
- Stainless bowl (large for draining)
- Large coffee filters or cheesecloth

Yields: 32 oz

Per Serving (1 cup): 24g, 24g, 8g = 96 + 96 + 72 = 264 calories

Directions:

1. Note: You must use non-homogenized yogurt, or the whey will not separate and you will end up with a soggy mess.

2. Line colander with coffee filters (they may have to overlap to get a good fit) or cheesecloth. Transfer yogurt from container to a colander and set into a stainless bowl for draining.

3. Cover the colander with plastic, and place everything in the refrigerator overnight. This will drain the whey out of the yogurt and leave you with a nice, firm yogurt cheese in the morning.

23. Potato Salad

~ For summer celebrations ~

Ingredients

- Potatoes, boiled and roughly chopped (3 Idaho or 6 red)
- Eggs, boiled and peeled (5)
- Celery (.75 c)
- Red onion (.25 c)
- Pickle relish (.25 c)
- Cider vinegar (1 T)
- Mayonnaise (.5 c)
- Mustard (1 tea)
- Sea salt and fresh ground pepper (to taste)
- Pinch of sugar (1 tea)
- Paprika
- Fresh parsley, chopped
- Green olives

Tools

- Stockpot with lid, 5-6 qt
- Colander
- Veggie knife
- Paring knife
- Chopping board
- Measuring cups and spoons
- Stainless bowl (large)

Serves: 6-8

Per Serving (1/8): 20g, 5g, 8g = 80 + 20 + 72 = 172 calories

Directions:

1. Scrub potatoes and place in a pan along with eggs, and fill the pan with water until covered. Place on high heat and cover. When the pot starts to boil, reduce heat so that it doesn't boil over. You want a high simmer. Remove eggs after 15 minutes. Check after 25 minutes for doneness; potatoes should be fork-tender.

2. When done, turn potatoes out in a colander and run under cold water to stop cooking. Cut potatoes into quarters to help with cooling. Set aside.

3. Chop celery and onion and place in a large bowl. Peel and chop eggs; add into the bowl with the celery. Cut potatoes into irregular bite-size pieces (don't make little cubes). Mix well.

4. To potato mixture, add relish, vinegar, mayo, mustard, salt, pepper, and sugar. Mix well and taste for seasoning. If flat, it might need a bit more mustard, vinegar, or salt. Add a little bit more, tasting after each addition.

5. Toss and top with paprika, parsley, and green olives. Cover in plastic and refrigerate at least 2 hours or overnight. The more it sits, the better it tastes.

24. Poppy Seed Dressing

~ Sweet and tangy ~

Ingredients

- Poppy seeds (1.5 T)
- Safflower oil (1 c)
- Onion, finely minced (1.5 T)
- White balsamic vinegar (.5 c)
- Sea salt (.25 tea)
- Dry mustard (1 tea)
- Sugar (.5 c)

Tools

- Veggie knife
- Measuring cup
- Measuring spoon
- Stainless mixing bowl
- Wisk
- Funnel (.25 - .3 inch opening, medium)
- Dressing carafe

Yields: 1.5 c - keeps refrigerated up to 2 weeks.

Per Serving (1 tablespoon): 6g, 0g, 9g = 24 + 0 + 81 = 105 calories

Directions:

1. In a bowl, whisk together sugar, dry mustard, salt, and vinegar. Gradually whisk in oil to create an emulsion or until vinegar and oil no longer separate. Stir in poppy seeds and onions.

2. Transfer to dressing carafe with a wide mouth or use a funnel for containers with a small opening.

25. Red Wine Vinaigrette

~ A pantry staple ~

Ingredients
- Red wine vinegar (1 c)
- Red wine, dry (.5 c)
- Sugar (dash)
- Oregano (.5 tea)
- Thyme (.25)
- Cumin (.25)
- Sea salt (.5 tea)
- Fresh ground pepper (.5 tea)
- Garlic, minced (2 cloves)
- Olive oil (.25 c)

Tools
- Stainless bowl (medium)
- Wisk
- Paring knife
- Salad dressing carafe

Yields: 1 cup
Per Serving (1 tablespoon): 0.5g, 0g, 3g = 2 + 0 +27 = 29 calories

Directions:

Combine vinegar, sugar, oregano, thyme, cumin, salt, pepper, and garlic. Whisk in olive oil (thin stream method) and transfer to the carafe. Keep refrigerated until use.

Chapter 7: Dinner

1. Baked Falafel

~ This reduced-fat version will soon be a favorite ~

Ingredients
- Olive oil (2 T)
- Egg, beaten (1)
- Flour (1 T)
- Baking soda (.25 tea)
- Salt (.25 tea)
- Ground coriander (.25 tea)
- Ground cumin (1 tea)
- Garlic, minced (3 cloves)
- Fresh parsley, chopped (.25 c)
- Garbanzo beans, rinsed and drained (1, 15oz can)
- Onion, chopped (.25 c)

Tools
- Food processor or potato masher
- Stainless bowl (large)
- Measuring cups and spoons
- Cast iron skillet (large)

Serves: 4
Per Serving (1/4): 29g, 8g, 9g = 116 + 32 + 81 = 229 calories

Directions:

1. Set oven to 400 degrees (F) and pre-heat.

2. Wrap chopped onion in a paper towel and squeeze out as much moisture as you can. Set aside.

3. If you have a food processor, add baking soda, salt, coriander, cumin, garlic, parsley, and garbanzo beans to the processor. Blend until mixture is coarsely pureed. Use a short blast of 4 seconds, so you don't get the mixture too smooth. Transfer to the large stainless mixing bowl when you are satisfied with the texture.

If you do not have a food processor, put the same ingredients in a large stainless mixing bowl and smash/blend with a potato masher.

4. Add onion to the bean mixture and blend well. Add egg and flour and stir well. Divide mixture into four portions and shape into large patties. Let stand for 15 minutes while the oven is heating.

5. In your large cast-iron skillet, heat olive oil with the burner on medium-high heat. Brown the bean patties on each side, approximately 3 minutes per side, until golden brown.

6. Place the skillet in the hot oven and bake until the patties are heated through, approximately 10 minutes.

Remember to use your oven mitt to remove the skillet!

Note: You can make smaller falafel, and use it as an appetizer. Or, you can make hummus falafel pita sandwiches or served as a side.

2. Lime Grilled Pork Tenderloin

~ *A great high-protein, low-fat choice* ~

Ingredients
- Cilantro leaves, loose (.5 c)
- Garlic, minced (1 clove)
- Ground cumin, (.5 tea)
- Sea salt and fresh ground pepper (to taste)
- Cider vinegar (2 T)
- Lime juice (.25 c - appr. 3 limes)
- Olive oil (3 T)
- Pork tenderloin, boneless (2 lb)

Tools
- Large Ziploc bag or air-tight container
- Paring knife
- Stainless bowl (small)
- Basting brush (small)
- Ramekin or glass bowl (small)
- Meat thermometer
- Meat tongs

Serves: 6
Per Serving (1/6): 2g, 40g, 12g = 8 + 160 + 108 = 276 calories

Directions:

1. Remove silverskin and excess fat from the tenderloin. Place in a Ziploc bag and pour in olive oil.

2. Whisk together vinegar, lime juice, garlic, cumin, salt, pepper, and cilantro leaves. Reserve about a tablespoon of the marinade in a ramekin for basting, and add 2 teaspoons of olive oil to

the marinade in a ramekin.

3. Pour remaining mixture over the tenderloin, and close Ziploc bag, squeezing out as much air as you can.

4. Set gas grill to medium or, if using charcoal, bank coals so that you are not cooking over direct heat. Place your tenderloin on the grill and discard bag with marinade. Only baste using the marinade you reserved in the ramekin.

5. Cook covered, turning every 2-3 minutes and basting with reserved marinade each turn. The meat has finished cooking when your meat thermometer reads 140 degrees. The tenderloin should be slightly pink but thoroughly cooked on the inside.

6. Take it off the grill and place on a clean, warm pan and cover with foil. Let rest for 10 minutes before slicing. Garnish serving platter with lime wedges and some sprigs of cilantro.

3. Greek Lemon Chicken With Herb Rice

~ If you have big eaters, you might want to double this recipe ~

Ingredients
- Sea salt (.5 tea)
- Garlic, minced (4 cloves)
- Oregano, dried (1 T)
- Lemon juice (4 T - 2 large)
- Lemon zest, from juiced lemons
- Olive oil (1 T)
- Chicken thighs, skin on and bone in (5)

Rice
- Fresh ground black pepper (to taste)
- Sea salt (.66 tea)
- Oregano, dried (2 tea)
- Ground thyme (.5 tea)
- Water (.66 c)
- Chicken stock (1.5 c)
- Lemon juice (4 T - 2 large)
- Lemon zest, from juiced lemons
- Brown rice (1 c)
- Onion, diced (1 small)
- Olive oil (1.5 T)

Tools
- Cast iron skillet (large)
- Ziploc bag (1 gal)
- Zester
- Foil

Serves: 5
Per Serving (1/5): 31g, 7g, 15g = 124 + 28 + 135 = 287 calories

Directions:

1. In a small, stainless bowl, whisk together salt, garlic, oregano, lemon juice, and lemon zest to make the marinade. Place chicken thighs in a large Ziploc bag and drizzle with olive oil. Pour the marinade over thighs. Let sit in the refrigerator for 20 minutes to 24 hrs.

2. Using a cast iron skillet, heat .5 olive oil to medium-high. While the pan is heating, preheat oven to 350 degrees.

3. Sear chicken in skillet, skin side down, until skin is golden and crispy (4-5 minutes). Turn chicken and repeat. Remove chicken from pan and set aside. Drain the fat from the pan into an empty can, not down the sink, and return pan to heat.

4. Saute onion in the remaining olive oil until translucent (3-4 minutes). Stir brown rice into onions and heat through (about 3 minutes). Stir in salt, pepper, oregano, and thyme. Then stir in the liquids: water, stock, lemon juice, and zest. Let the mixture simmer for 30 seconds.

5. Place the chicken thighs on top and put a lid on the pan (or foil if there is no lid). Bake in the oven for 35 minutes. Remove cover and back for another 10 minutes, or until all the liquid has been absorbed. Rice should be tender.

6. Remove skillet from the oven and let rest for 10 minutes. Garnish with fresh parsley and lemon zest.

4. Stuffed Onions

~ *This is a make-today-serve-tomorrow dish* ~

Ingredients
- Eggs, lightly beaten (2 large)
- Pine nuts, toasted (.3 c)
- Hard Romano cheese, grated (.5 c - or parmesan)
- Crushed red pepper flakes (pinch)
- Tomato paste (1 T), dissolved in warm water (2 T)
- Red wine, dry (.5 c)
- Bulgur wheat, cooked (.66 c)
- Fresh dill, chopped (1 c)
- Lean ground pork or beef (10 oz)
- Garlic, minced (2 cloves)
- Olive oil (.25 c)
- Sea salt (to taste)
- Onions, unpeeled (6 medium)

Sauce
- Fresh parsley, chopped (3 T)
- Sea salt and fresh ground pepper
- Chicken stock or water (.5 c)
- Red wine, dry (.25 c)
- Dried oregano, crumbled (1 tea)
- Bay leaf, broken up (1)
- Grated ripe tomatoes, or canned diced tomatoes with juice (2 c)
- Olive oil (.25 c)

Tools
- Large stock pot
- Paring knife
- Colander

- Large stainless skillet
- Baking dish (13 x9)
- Pam cooking spray or lightly brush with oil

Serves: 6
Per Serving (1/6): 35g, 26g, 29g = 140 + 104 + 261 = 505 calories

Directions:

1. In a large stock pot, bring water to a boil. Rinse unpeeled onions, and cut a slit on the side of each onion that cuts from top to bottom, halfway through the onion. Place the onions in the boiling water and add 2 tea of sea salt. Simmer over medium heat for 25 minutes until soft.

2. Using a slotted spoon, transfer onions to a colander and rinse under cold water to halt the cooking. Allow to drain and cool.

3. Slice off the top and bottom of onions, and peel off the skin and second layer (more if they are tough). Squeeze the center of the onion out and set aside. There should be 2-3 layers of the onion; gently separate these and set aside. Onions can be cooked and separated up to two days earlier. Cover with plastic wrap and store in the refrigerator.

4. Chop the onion centers you set aside earlier. Saute in a large skillet using the .25 cup olive oil for 3 minutes until onions are soft. Add the garlic cloves and saute for another 2 minutes. Add meat and cook until there's no pink meat. Stir in dill, pepper flakes, bulgur, wine, and tomato paste mixture. Mix thoroughly and remove from heat. Stir in salt, pepper, cheese, and pine nuts.

5. Allow mixture to cool slightly (you don't want the eggs to cook when you stir them into the meat mixture. Taste the mixture, and adjust seasoning if needed, then stir in eggs.

6. Set your oven to 400 degrees. Stuff the onion skins with about 2 tablespoons of stuffing. Roll the onion skin closed (skin should wrap around stuffing), and place seam side down in lightly oiled or sprayed baking pan. Don't forget to grease sides of the pan.

7. Heat olive oil in a skillet over medium-high setting and saute tomatoes, bay leaf, and oregano for 5 minutes or until sauce begins to thicken. Remove from heat, and add wine and chicken stock or water. Stir and pour over stuffed onions, then sprinkle with salt and pepper, to taste.

8. Place onion dish in the oven, and reduce the heat to 375 degrees. Bake for 45 minutes, basting onions with the sauce every 7-10 minutes. When onions are soft and the sauce has thickened, the dish is ready.

9. Remove from oven and let cool. Store in refrigerator until ready to use (could be frozen and served another week. It must be in an oven-proof dish, such as CorningWare if frozen. To reheat, place the dish in a hot oven (375 degrees) and reheat until the dish is hot all the way through. Do not thaw dish first.

10. Garnish with parsley and serve.

" Are you enjoying this book? If so, I'd be really happy if you could leave a short review on Amazon, it means a lot to me! Thank you."

5. Greek-Style Grouper

~ Another hometown favorite ~

Ingredients
- Skinless grouper fillets (4, 6-7oz)
- Olive oil (2 T)
- Sea salt and fresh ground pepper (to taste)
- Lemon juice (.5 lemon to squeeze)
- Oregano, crumbled (1 tea, 4 pinches)
- Paprika (pinch)

Garnish
- Lemon wedges (4)
- Parsley, chopped (1 T)

Tools
- Large skillet, nonstick, oven-safe
- Spatula
- Measuring spoons

Serves: 4
Per Serving (1/4): 0g, 42g, 9g = 0 + 168 + 81 = 249 calories

Directions:
1. In a skillet, heat oil over high heat. Sprinkle grouper fillets generously with salt, a pinch of pepper, and oregano. Place fillets in the pan, and reduce heat to medium. Cook for 2 minutes on the stove top.
2. Sprinkle tops of fillets with paprika and drizzle with olive oil. Transfer skillet to the oven for 6 minutes or until fillets are just cooked through. Meat should be glistening and tender and slide away in flakes.

3. Garnish with chopped parsley and a lemon wedge. Serve immediately.

6. Broiled Snapper

~ For candlelight and flowers ~

Ingredients
- Red snapper (1.5 lb) - ask your fishmonger to fillet and save the head and bone portion for you.
- Olive oil (1 T)
- Oregano, dried (1 tea)
- Paprika
- Sea salt (to taste)

Tools
- Foil-lined baking sheet (2)
- Pam cooking spray or oil
- Spatula

Serves: 4
Per Serving (1/4): 0g, 45g, 6g = 0 + 180 + 54 = 234 calories

Directions:

1. Spray two foil-lined baking sheets with cooking spray or brush with safflower oil. Set oven rack 4-6 inches from heat and turn the oven on broil.

2. On the first pan, put the snapper head and backbone portion and spray with cooking spray. There is quite a bit of good meat that most people leave at the fish market. They charge quite a bit for snapper cheeks.

3. Place snapper fillets on the second pan (skin side down), and sprinkle salt to taste, paprika, and oregano, crushing as you go. Drizzle with olive oil and put under the broiler for 8-10 minutes or until the fish is opaque and just cooked through.

4. Garnish with a lemon wedge and serve immediately.

Note: When the snapper has finished cooking, adjust the oven to bake at 350 degrees, and put it in the pan with the head on it. Set your timer for 5 minutes; you might have to cover the backbone with foil to keep it from drying out. The fish should be done when the snapper throat flesh is opaque and the eyes look cooked. If you don't want to pick the meat for a salad or appetizer, you can at least pick it clean for your four-legged friends.

7. Pan-Broiled Chicken Breast

~ Leftovers make a great high-protein snack ~

Ingredients
- Chicken breast, skinless, boneless (2)
- Olive oil (2 T)
- Sea salt and ground pepper (to taste)
- Ground thyme (1 tea)
- Dill weed, dry (1 tea)
- Lemon, half

Tools
- Cast iron skillet (large)
- Meat tongs
- Measuring spoons
- Meat thermometer

Serves: 4
Per Serving (1/4): 0g, 71g, 15g = 0 + 284 + 135 = 419 calories

Directions:

1. Heat skillet over medium-high heat and add oil.

2. Season chicken breast with salt, pepper, thyme, and dill. I like to use the shaker top with the thyme and dill rather than measure it out and dredge or rub. With the shaker, I get a light and even coverage.

Tip: Leave the chicken on the packaging it came in and shake on season and herbs. Transfer the chicken to pan, season side down. Now, shake the season and herbs onto the exposed side.

3. Sear chicken for 2-3 minutes each side then turn down the heat to medium or medium-low. Cook on each side for 10 minutes or until a meat thermometer reads 165. Chicken should look plump and juicy.

4. Let rest at least 7 minutes prior to slicing. Slice chicken into one-inch diagonal pieces, and transfer equal portions to each plate.

It may be served on top of Tropical Salad: Fruit, Nuts & More in lieu of bacon. I suggest the Lemon Mustard Dressing or with roasted potatoes and steamed asparagus.

Change it up by using the spice rub.

8. Grilled Lamb & Fig Kebabs

~ *This dish is a wondrous mix of flavors to be savored* ~

Ingredients
- Green onions, trimmed and cut into 1.5 in pieces (6 - thick)
- Fresh ground pepper (1 tea)
- Sea salt (2 tea)
- Ground coriander (2 tea)
- Ground cumin (1 T + 1 tea)
- Garlic, minced (2 T, 3-4 cloves)
- Olive oil (.25 c)
- Black Mission figs or Brown Turkey figs (12-14 halved lengthwise through the stem - look for firm ripe figs. If they are overripe, they will fall off the skewers)
- Leg of lamb, boneless, trimmed, cut into 1.5-inch cubes (3.5 lbs)

Glaze
- Fresh mint leaves, finely chopped (.25 c + extra for garnish)
- Lemon zest (from 1 lemon)
- Crushed red pepper flakes (2 tea)
- Red wine vinegar (.3 c)
- Apricot preserves or jam (.66 c)

Tools
- Metal skewers, 17 inches (8-10)
- Small saucepan
- Stainless bowl (large)
- Plastic cutting board, for meat
- Zester
- Measuring cups and spoons
- Basting brush (small)

Serves: 6-8
Per Serving (1/8): 40g, 58g, 21g = 160 + 232 + 189 = 581 calories

Directions:

1. Glaze: Combine apricot jam, vinegar, lemon zest, and pepper flakes in a small saucepan. Over high heat, bring the mixture to a boil, then reduce heat to simmer. Stir occasionally for 6-8 minutes or until mixture thickens to a jam consistency. Remove from heat and let cool for 5-10 minutes before stirring in mint.

2. Slice lamb into 1.5-inch cubes and place in a large bowl. Add figs and gently toss with olive oil, salt, pepper, garlic, cumin, and coriander. Marinade while starting the grill.

3. If using charcoal, you want the heat to be one briquette thick. If on a gas grill, preheat to medium-high.

4. Thread lamb cubes, figs, and green onion (through center width on both fig and onion). After the third fig, end with a cube of lamb.

5. Place skewers on the grill and cook 4 minutes with the cover on. Brush liberally with glaze and turn. Grill covered for 3 more minutes. Glaze and turn. Grill another half minute with the cover off for medium-rare lamb. The lamb will continue to cook when removed from heat. Rest for 5 minutes.

6. You can serve on kebabs, but I prefer to slide contents onto a large warm platter, keeping the line of the kebab. It's easier for your guest, and no one gets burned. Garnish with extra mint sprinkled on top and wedges of lemon.

9. Chicken Pitas

~ Yum ... yum ... yum ~

Ingredients
- Fresh ground pepper (to taste)
- Sea salt (.25 tea)
- Garlic (1 clove pressed)
- Lemon juice (1 tea)
- Greek yogurt, plain (.66 c)

- Chicken thighs, boneless, skinless (4)
- Turmeric (.25 tea)
- Fresh ground pepper (.5 tea)
- Sea salt (.5 tea)
- Paprika (1 tea)
- Ground cumin (1 tea)
- Garlic, pressed (3 cloves)
- Lemon juice (3 T)
- Olive oil (.25 c)

- Tomato, chopped (1 large)
- Cucumber, chopped (1 medium)
- Romaine, shredded (4-5 leaves)
- Pita bread (4 loaves)
- Chicken broth or water (.25 c)
- Red onion, cut into wedges (1 small)

Tools
- Stainless bowl (2, small)
- Skillet, nonstick (medium)
- Meat tongs
- Meat thermometer

Serves: 4
Per Servings (1/4): 9g, 92g, 31g = 36 + 368 + 279 = 683 calories

Directions:

1. Combine lemon juice, garlic, cumin, paprika, salt, pepper, and turmeric in a small bowl and mix. Place thighs in Ziploc and coat with olive oil. Pour lemon marinade over thighs. Close up the bag and press out as much air as possible. Marinate in refrigerator 20 minutes up to 2 hours.

2. Combine yogurt, lemon juice, garlic, salt, and pepper. Mix until yogurt and lemon juice do not separate.

3. Set your oven to 250 degrees for warming.

4. Remove chicken thighs from marinade and (discard bag with marinade) place in a nonstick skillet over medium-high heat. Sear for 2-4 minutes until golden brown. Turn thighs and cook for another 2-4 minutes. Test with a meat thermometer for an internal temperature of 165 degrees. Continue to cook and turn the meat until the thickest part of the thigh reads 165 degrees. You may need to turn down the heat if the thighs start to brown too much.

5. Remove from heat when done. Place on a plate and cover with foil to keep the meat warm.

6. Return heat to medium-high and deglaze pan with .25 cup chicken broth or water, scraping the bottom of the pan while the liquid simmers. You want all of that goodie sticking to the pan to come loose. Add onions to the pan.

7. Put your pita bread in foil and place in the oven while the onions cook.

8. Continue to cook onions until they reach the desired level of softness for 4-10 minutes and remove from heat.

9. Remove pita from the oven. Slice thighs into strips, and place them in warm pita loaves. Top with sautéed onions, lettuce, tomato, cucumbers, and yogurt.

10. Mediterranean Shrimp Fajitas

~ *A tasty treat for any occasion* ~

Ingredients
- Tortillas, warmed (1 package 6" yellow corn)
- Fresh cilantro, loose leaf
- Lime (1)
- Smoked paprika (.5 tea)
- Ground cumin (.5 tea)
- Yellow onion, minced (1 small)
- Garlic, smashed and minced (2 cloves)
- Chili powder (.5 tea)
- Fresh ground pepper (to taste)
- Sea salt (1 tea)
- Olive oil (1.5 T)
- Red onion, sliced (1 small)
- Orange, red and yellow bell pepper, thinly sliced (1 each, small)
- Shrimp, peeled and deveined (1.5 lbs)

Tools
- Stainless bowl (large)
- Cookie sheet (large)
- Cooking spray
- Veggie knife
- Shrimp deveiner

Serves: 4
Per Serving (1/4 with 2 tortillas): 35g, 43g, 10g = 140 + 172 + 90 = 402 calories

Directions:

1. Set oven to 450 degrees.

2. Combine and toss paprika, cumin, onion, garlic, chili powder, salt, pepper, olive oil, red onion, bell pepper, and shrimp in large bowl.

3. Prepare a baking sheet with nonstick cooking spray.

4. Spread shrimp and veggie mixture on a baking sheet.

5. Bake in the oven for 8 minutes at 450 degrees. Switch setting to broil and cook 2 more minutes or until the shrimp is opaque or cooked through. Remove from the oven.

6. Transfer fajita mixture to a serving platter, and squeeze lime juice over the shrimp and veggies and top with fresh cilantro. Serve with warm tortillas and cold beer.

11. Spicy Pan-Seared Salmon

~ A quick, zesty change to grilled lemon & dill ~

Ingredients
- Lemon zest (1 tea)
- Cayenne pepper (pinch)
- Fresh ground pepper (.25 tea)
- Sea salt (.25 tea)
- Ground coriander (.5 tea)
- Ground cumin (.5 tea)
- Onion, minced (2 tea)
- Garlic, crushed, minced (1 tea)
- Paprika (1 tea)
- Safflower oil (2 T)
- Salmon fillets, skinned (4, roughly 1.24 - 1.5 lbs)

Tools
- Stainless bowl (large)
- Cast iron skillet (large)
- Veggie knife

Serves: 4
Per Serving (1/4): 0g, 33g, 17g = 0 + 132 + 153 = 285 calories

Directions:

1. In a bowl, place fillets and drizzle with 2 tablespoons oil. Sprinkle fillets evenly with salt, pepper, cayenne, coriander, cumin, onion, garlic, paprika, and lemon zest. Toss fillets gently to coat with herbs and oil evenly. Let salmon fillets marinate for 20 minutes to 24 hours (if preparing a day ahead).

2. Over medium-high heat, place skillet and add 2-3 tablespoons of oil. Add fillets to hot pan and sear for 4 minutes or until golden brown. Gently turn fillets and sear for another 4 minutes. Remove from the heat and transfer to a serving platter.

Serve with Salsa Fresca and Toasty Couscous.

12. Greek Flank Steak

~ Have a glass of wine with this dinner ~

Ingredients
- Oregano, dried (1 tea)
- Fresh mint, chopped (2 T)
- Dijon mustard (1 T)
- Red wine vinegar (.25 c)
- Lemon zest (1 T)
- Soy sauce (.25 c)
- Lemon juice (.25 c)
- Olive oil (3 T)
- Flank steak (2 lbs)

Tools
- Baking dish (9x9)
- Stainless bowl (medium)
- Wisk

Serves: 4-6
Per Serving (1/6): 1g, 43g, 21g = 4 + 172 + 189 = 365 calories

Directions:

1. Combine oregano, mint, Dijon mustard, vinegar, zest, soy sauce, and lemon juice in a bowl. Whisk in oil poured in a thin stream. Reserve .25 cup of marinade for basting.

2. Place flank steak in a glass dish and cover completely with soy sauce mixture. Marinade for 8 to 24 hours.

3. Grill over offset heat (if using charcoal) or medium for gas grill. Grill meat for 5-8 minutes per side. Baste meat with reserved marinade while cooking. Meat should read at least 145 degrees for rare at 5 minutes per side.

4. Let steak sit for at least 5 minutes. Slice on the diagonal against the grain or cuts will be tough.

5. Serve hot with Tzatziki and Greek Salad (omit shrimp unless you are planning a big surf and turf dinner).

13. Mediterranean Stuffed Peppers

~ *A fiesta for the eyes and taste buds* ~

Ingredients
- Chicken broth or water (.75 c)
- Bell Peppers, mixed color, tops removed, and cored (6)
- Water (2.25 c)
- Tomato sauce (3 T)
- Paprika (.5 tea)
- Bulgur wheat (1 c) soaked in water for 15 min then drained
- Parsley, chopped (.5 c + garnish)
- Chickpeas, cooked or canned (1 c)
- Garlic, crushed, minced (1 clove)
- Ground allspice (.5 tea)
- Sea salt and fresh ground pepper (to taste)
- Ground beef (.5 lb)
- Yellow onion, chopped (1 small)
- Olive oil

Tools
- Saucepan (medium)
- Wooden spoon
- Cookie sheet covered with foil
- Cooking spray
- Paper bag
- Round or oval baking dish (9x9ish)

Serves: 6
Per Serving (1/6): 35g, 19g, 6g = 140 + 76 + 54 = 270 calories

Directions:

1. Heat 1 tablespoon oil in a saucepan. Add onions and saute over medium heat until golden.

Add ground beef and cook until no pink meat is left. Stir in allspice, garlic, and season, to taste, then add chickpeas and let cook for 2 minutes.

2. To the same mixture, add bulgur wheat, tomato sauce, paprika, and parsley. Stir in 2.25 cups of water and bring to boil. Reduce heat to low and cover for 10-20 minutes. Check to make sure bulgur is not scorching.

3. While the filling is cooking, put peppers on a foil-covered and sprayed cookie sheet. Place under the broiler (4-6 inches from heat) for 10-15 minutes. Turn peppers so that each side gets charred. Allow only the skin to char, not the meat of the pepper. When all sides have blistered and charred, remove from the oven and put in a paper bag to cool. This helps the skin to sweat, which makes the peppers easier to peel.

4. Change oven setting from broil to bake at 350 degrees.

5. Remove filling from the heat. The mixture should be done, and all liquid should be absorbed into bulgur. If not, let it sit covered for 10 minutes.

6. Spray baking dish with cooking spray and place peppers, open side up in the dish. Spoon enough meat filling into each pepper, fill to the top. Pour .75 cup chicken broth or water into the bottom of the baking dish, around the peppers.

7. Cover snuggly with foil and bake for 20-30 minutes.

8. Take the baking dish from the oven and garnish with parsley. Serve hot with salad and side of Tzatziki or plain Greek yogurt.

This is also good for freezing.

14. Arugula Shrimp Salad With White Beans

~ *Basil, shrimp, and cannellini* ~

Ingredients
- Baby arugula leaves (2 c)
- Lemon zest (.75 tea)
- Salt and pepper (to taste)
- Red onion, finely diced (.5 c)
- Grape tomatoes, halved (1 c)
- Cannellini white beans, rinsed and drained (2 15-oz cans)
- Olive oil (2 T)
- Shrimp, shelled and deveined (1 lb medium)
- Basil leaves, loose
- Red Wine Dressing

Tools
- Cast iron skillet (large)
- Spatula
- Stainless bowls (1 large, 1 medium)

Serves: 4
Per Serving (1/4): 23g, 34g, 9g = 92 + 136 + 81 = 309 calories

Directions:

1. Over high heat, add 2 tablespoons of olive oil to a large skillet. Wait until pan and oil are hot then add half the shrimp at a time and saute about a minute on each side until opaque. Transfer the first batch to a medium bowl and repeat on the second half of shrimp.
2. While the shrimps are cooling, combine beans, tomatoes, red onion, zest, and season to taste. Add shrimp, arugula leaves, and .25 cup of Red Wine Dressing (shaken well) and mix gently.
3. Divide onto four plates and garnish with basil leaves.

15. Quick Mediterranean Chicken Pasta

~ Try the Pan-Broiled Chicken Breast in this ~

Ingredients
- Sea salt and pepper (to taste)
- Lemon juice (1 T)
- Feta cheese, crumbled (4 oz)
- Kalamata olives, sliced (3.5 oz)
- Oregano, dried (.25 tea)
- Fresh basil leaves, light chop (6 leaves)
- Chicken breast, cooked, chopped (10 oz, or 2 breasts)
- Grape tomatoes, halved (1 c)
- Olive oil (2 T)
- Penne pasta (12 oz)

Serves: 6-8
Per Serving (1/6): 34g, 19g, 13g = 136 + 76 + 117 = 329 calories

Directions:

1. Cook pasta according to directions on the package and set aside in a large bowl to cool.

2. Add and mix well the chicken, tomatoes, basil, olives, feta, and oregano. Add lemon juice and season to taste. Stir well and taste; adjust seasoning as you like.

Serve immediately or cover with plastic to serve at a later time.

16. Baked Greek Salmon in a Pouch

~ Five ingredients! Quick and delicious ~

Ingredients
- Feta cheese, crumbled (8 T)
- Grape tomatoes, halved (1 pint)
- Onion, chopped (1 medium)
- Pesto (.5 c)
- Salmon fillets (4-6oz)

Tools
- Cookie sheet
- Foil sheets (4, large enough to wrap salmon and topping)
- Veggie knife
- Cooking spray

Serves: 4
Per Serving (1/4): 9g + 40g + 28g = 36 + 160 + 252 = 448 calories

Directions:

1. While heating the oven to 350 degrees, spray large pieces of aluminum foil with cooking spray.

2. Place the fillet in the middle of each sheet of foil. Top salmon with pesto, onion, tomatoes, and feta crumbles.

3. Create little tents by folding the foil together over the middle of the salmon, leaving room for steam, then pinch sides together. Bake for 25 minutes. The fish should flake easily when done.

17. Tzatziki

~ *Great dipping sauce at snack time* ~

Ingredients
- Sea salt (1 tea)
- Garlic, crushed, minced (1 clove)
- Fresh mint, chopped (2 T)
- Fresh dill, chopped (2 T)
- Cucumber, chopped fine (.5 c)
- Lemon juice (.25 c)
- Greek yogurt, plain (.75 c)

Tools
- Stainless bowl (medium)
- Veggie knife
- Wisk

Serves: 4-6
Per Serving (1/6): 3g + 2g + .5g = 12 + 8 + 4.5 = 24.5 calories

Directions:

1. Whisk together salt, garlic, mint, dill, and lemon juice. Stir in cucumber and yogurt until liquid is incorporated into the yogurt. Taste and adjust for seasoning.

18. Toasty Couscous

~ Nutty goodness ~

Ingredients
- Parsley, chopped (1 T)
- Garlic, smashed, minced (1 clove)
- Olive oil (1 T)
- Sea salt (to taste)
- Water (1.25 c)
- Couscous (1 c)

Tools
- Saucepan, nonstick (medium)
- Wooden spoon
- Stainless bowl (medium)

Serves: 4
Per Serving (1/4): 34g, 6g, 4g = 136 + 24 + 36 = 196 calories

Directions:

1. With the saucepan over medium heat, add couscous and toast for a minute or two. You will want to shake the pan or stir the couscous while toasting to avoid burning. Pour into a bowl and set aside.

2. Using the same saucepan, bring water to a boil. Add salt (to taste), olive oil, and garlic. Pour in the couscous and stir. Turn off the heat, and cover the pan with lid. Let sit for 5-7 minutes. Transfer to a serving bowl; add parsley and toss. Serve warm.

19. Salsa Fresca

~Kalamata olives, yellow bell pepper, & fresh dill ~

Ingredients
- Sea salt and fresh ground pepper (to taste)
- Lemon juice (1 tea)
- Lemon zest (.5 tea)
- Fresh parsley (1 tea)
- Fresh dill (1 tea)
- Red onion, chopped (2 T)
- Kalamata olives, diced (2 T)
- Yellow bell pepper, finely diced (1/4 of pepper)
- Cucumber, finely diced (1 small)
- Grape tomatoes, halved (1 c)

Tools
- Veggie knife
- Zester
- Stainless bowl (small)

Serves: 4
Per Serving (1/4): 6g, 1g, 1g = 24 + 4 + 9 = 37 calories

Directions:

Combine tomatoes, cucumber, bell pepper, olives, onion, dill, and parsley in a small bowl and mix well. Add zest, lemon juice, salt, and pepper, to taste. Mix well. Serve right away or cover with plastic and store in the refrigerator until ready to serve.

20. Chicken Spice Rub

~ *Another one for the pantry* ~

Ingredients
- Paprika (4 T)
- Turmeric (2 T)
- Curry (3 tea)
- White pepper (1 tea)
- Chili powder (2 T)
- Cumin (1 tea)
- Thyme (.5 tea)
- Sea salt (.5 tea)
- Cheyanne pepper (.5)
- Fresh ground black pepper (.5)
- Dry English mustard (1 tea)

Tools
- Measuring spoons
- Metal spice shaker

Directions:

1. Using a screw-top metal shaker, add all the ingredients and mix together using a fork. Blend well. This rub keeps well in the shaker and is easy to use on various cuts of meat if you want a bit of spice in your life.

Chapter 8: Desserts

1. Vegan No-Bake Cookies

~ Cinnamon, brown sugar, & oats ~

Ingredients

- Sea salt (pinch)
- Vanilla extract (1 tea)
- Ground cinnamon (1 tea)
- Rolled oats (1.66 c)
- Skim milk (.25 c)
- Coconut oil (.25 c)
- Brown sugar, packed (.3 c)
- Almond butter or natural peanut butter (.75 c)

Tools

- Saucepan (medium)
- Wooden spoon
- Large metal spoon
- Cookie sheet
- Parchment paper

Serves: 22
Per Serving (1): 8g, 3g, 7g = 32 + 12 + 63 = 107 calories

Directions:

1. In a medium saucepan, heat almond or peanut butter, brown sugar, coconut oil, and milk. Stir over medium heat until the sugar has dissolved and everything is blended smoothly. Remove from heat. To this mixture add salt, vanilla, cinnamon, and stir in oats and let sit for 5 minutes.

2. Using a large spoon, drop about a tablespoonful of dough onto a parchment paper lined baking sheet (you may use wax paper or plastic wrap). Press into 2-inch circles and refrigerate until firm (2 hours).

Will keep up to five days in the refrigerator in an airtight container.

2. Yogurt Cheese Cake

~ Creamy mango & cherry swirl ~

Ingredients

- Yogurt cheese (2 c)
- Stevia (3 T)
- Sugar or honey (3 T)
- Cornstarch (1 T)
- Lemon juice (1 T)
- Vanilla (1 tea)
- Eggs (2)
- Mangos, pitted (1 c)
- Fresh Bing cherries, stemmed and pitted (1 c)
- Whole cherries and mint leaves for garnish

Tools

- Large springform pan
- Cooking spray
- Food processor
- Stainless bowls (2 medium)
- Stainless bowls (2 small)

Serves: 10-12

Per Serving (1/10): 15g, 6g, 3g = 60 + 24 + 27 = 111 calories

Directions:

1. Set your oven to 325 degrees and heat. Process mango flesh in a food processor until smooth. Pour into a small bowl and set aside. Do the same for the Bing cherries and set aside (do not mix the two).

2. Combine yogurt cheese, stevia, sugar, cornstarch, lemon juice, vanilla, and eggs and mix until smooth.

3. Pour half batter into the other medium bowl; you should have equal parts per bowl. Add the mango to one bowl and the cherries to the other, and mix fruit in thoroughly.

4. Spray a springform pan with cooking spray and pour mango batter into one side and cherry batter into the other side of the pan. Gently take a knife and swirl from the cherry side into the mango and back around to give swirl design.

5. Bake for 40-50 minutes or until the inserted knife comes out clean. Let it cool to room temperature. Loosen the sides with a knife and then pop the springform to remove sides of the pan. Refrigerate 4 hours before serving.

6. Garnish with cherries and mint.

3. Luscious Baked Pears

~ Sweet and elegant ~

Ingredients

- Plain Greek yogurt
- Pecan Granola (.5 c)
- Vanilla extract (1 tea)
- Ground cinnamon (.25 tea)
- Maple syrup (.5 c)
- Anjou pears (4)

Tools

- Cookie sheet, sprayed or lined with parchment.
- Paring knife
- Fork (for whisking and drizzle)
- Small bowl for syrup

Serves: 4

Per Serving (1/4): 86g, 8g, 20g = 344 + 32 + 180 = 556 calories

Directions:

1. Set oven to 375 degrees. Prepare a baking sheet or a small metal pan with sides.

2. With a paring knife, halve and seed pears (you can use a melon baller or a teaspoon to remove seeds, if that is easier). Cut a small sliver off the rounded underside of pear to help them lay flat in the pan.

3. Place pears in the pan, cut side up, and sprinkle with cinnamon.

4. With a fork, whisk together maple syrup and vanilla. Drizzle all but 2 tablespoons of the mixture over the pears. The remaining syrup will be used for garnish.

5. Bake for 25 minutes. Pears should be soft, slightly brown at the edges, and fork-tender. Remove from the oven and drizzle with the remaining syrup mixture.

6. Serve warm with Pecan Granola in the center and a dollop of yogurt on the side.

4. Funky Monkey Yogurt

~ Bananas, peanuts, & peanut butter ~

Ingredients

- Vanilla extract (1 tea)
- Ground nutmeg (1 tea)
- Flaxseed meal (.25 c)
- Natural peanut butter, creamy (.5 c)
- Bananas, sliced (2 medium)
- Peanuts, roasted, chopped (1 c)
- Greek yogurt (4 c)

Tools

- Microwave safe ramekin (small)
- Stainless bowl (medium)
- Dessert bowls (8)

Serves: 8

Per Serving (1/8): 29g, 23g, 33g = 116 + 92 + 297 = 505 calories

Directions:

1. Combine yogurt, vanilla, and chopped peanuts in mixing bowl. Divide mixture evenly into dessert bowls and top with banana slices.

2. Melt peanut butter in the microwave for 30-40 seconds. Drizzle one tablespoon of peanut butter over each bowl, making flowery swirls over the bananas.

3. Sprinkle with nutmeg and flax seed and serve.

5. Raspberry Cream Cups

~ *Coconut, cashews, & maple syrup* ~

Ingredients

- Sea salt (pinch)
- Vanilla extract (2 tea)
- Lemon juice (.25 c and 2 tea)
- Fresh raspberries, room temperature (3 c). If using frozen berries, you will need 4 cups, and make sure to thaw to room temperature - no cold berries!
- Maple syrup (.5 c and 1 T)
- Coconut cream (.25 c). This is the top of full-fat coconut milk that has been refrigerated overnight. Open with a can opener and skim off the cream.
- Raw coconut oil (.75 c)
- Roasted cashews (1.5 c). Soak in boiling water (bring water to boil, remove from the stove, and add cashews). Let stand for an hour then drain.

- Sea salt (pinch)
- Vanilla extract (1 tea)
- Maple syrup (1.5 T)
- Roasted cashews, salted (1 c)
- Unsweetened coconut, shredded (.5 c)

Tools

- Saucepan (small and medium)
- Stainless bowls (medium)
- Muffin tin (12 cups + 2 small ramekins)
- Food processor
- Wooden spoon

- Cupcake liners

Serves: 14 cupcakes

Per Serving (1 cupcake): 25g, 4g, 25g = 100 + 16 + 225 = 341 calories

Directions:

1. Line muffin tin with cupcake liners.

2. In a small, thick-bottomed pan, heat shredded coconut flakes over medium-high heat, stirring frequently. You want a nice golden brown color, but coconut burns quickly, so watch it closely. When toasted, place into a bowl to cool for 5 minutes.

3. In a food processor, combine a pinch of salt, 1 teaspoon vanilla, 1.5 tablespoon of maple syrup, roasted cashews (not the ones that were soaked), and toasted coconut. Pulse until the mixture starts to clump and stick together. Do not process into a paste. Hint: when you pinch mixture between fingers it should stick and hold. If not, add a teaspoon of water, pulse, and test.

4. Press crust into the bottom of cupcake liners and place muffin tin in the refrigerator while making the filling.

5. Whip processor bowl clean as we will use it again for filling.

6. In a medium saucepan, add soaked cashews, coconut oil, coconut cream, remaining maple syrup, raspberries, lemon juice, remaining vanilla, and a pinch of salt. Heat over medium heat until the mixture is warmed and the coconut cream and oil are melted.

7. Pour the filling into a food processor and blend for 30-60 seconds until mixture is smooth (except for raspberry seeds).

8. Pour final filling mixture into each muffin cup (about .25 c). Pour any remaining filling into ramekins. Refrigerate for 6 hours or until firm. Cups may be stored in the freezer in an airtight container. Allow up to 3 hours to thaw in the refrigerator or 1.5 hours at room temperature.

6. Grecian Cinnamon Apple Cake

~ Olive oil, brown sugar, raisins, & walnuts ~

Ingredients

- Sesame seeds (3 T)
- Ground cinnamon (1.5 tea)
- Raisins (.5 c)
- Walnuts, chopped (.5 c)
- Apples, peeled, halved, cored, and thinly sliced (4) Granny Smith, Honey crisp, or Jonathans are good for baking.
- Vanilla extract (1 tea)
- Baking powder (2 tea)
- Wheat flour (2.5 c)
- Skim milk (1 c)
- Olive oil (1 c)
- Brown sugar (1 c + 2 T for topping)
- Eggs (4)

Tools

- Wooden spoon
- Stainless bowl (2, large)
- Measuring cups and spoons
- Wisk
- 9x9x3 cake pan, greased (cooking spray) and floured

Serves: 12

Per Serving (1/12): 50g, 7g, 23 = 200 + 28 + 207 = 435 calories

Directions:

1. Set oven to 375 degrees. Grease baking pan with either olive oil or cooking spray. Flour bottom and sides with 2 tablespoons of flour, and knock out excess flour.

2. Whisk eggs and sugar together until lightly blended. Whisk in olive oil in a thin stream until all oil is added.

3. Stir in milk and vanilla. Add all baking powder and wheat flour (.5 cup at a time) and fold in gently with a wooden spoon.

4. In a large bowl, combine apples, the remaining 2 tablespoons of sugar, cinnamon, walnuts, and raisins. Mix well to coat apples evenly with sugar and cinnamon.

5. Pour half cake batter into the pan. Gently spoon apple mixture onto the batter; cover evenly. Pour the remaining batter onto the apple mixture and sprinkle with sesame seeds on top.

6. Bake for 45-50 minutes or until a knife comes out clean. Let cool for 5 minutes. Run a knife along the edge to loosen, if needed. Place serving platter over the top and flip. If the cake did not come away, you may need to shake once.

7. Mediterranean Mousse

~ Honey & dark chocolate, that's no Bullwinkle ~

Ingredients

- Vanilla extract (.5 tea)
- Honey or maple syrup (1 T)
- Greek yogurt (2 c)
- Dark chocolate, semi-sweet, shaved or chopped fine (3.5 oz)
- Skim milk (.75 c)

Tools

- Saucepan (medium)
- Wooden spoon
- Stainless bowl (large)

Serves: 4

Per Serving (1/4): 28g, 9g, 10g = 112 + 36 + 90 = 238

Directions:

1. Combine milk and chocolate in a saucepan over medium heat. Stir constantly until the chocolate melts. Do not let the milk boil or the chocolate to scorch. When the chocolate has melted into the milk, add honey and vanilla. Mix well.

2. Remove from heat and set aside for a minute.

3. Spoon yogurt into a bowl. Spoon about .5 cup of yogurt into the chocolate milk and mix well. This will cool the milk down quicker. Now, pour the entire amount of chocolate mixture into the yogurt, and gently fold the chocolate into it.

4. Spoon chocolate yogurt mixture into dessert bowls, ramekins, or parfait glasses.

5. Chill in the refrigerator for 2 hours. Serve with a dollop of yogurt and a few fresh raspberries.

Chapter 9: Snacks and Sides

~ Sweet & savory pick-me-ups for any time of the day ~

1. Sweet Potatoes with Sesame Sauce

Ingredients

- Tahini, runny (2 T)
- Sea salt and fresh ground pepper (to taste)
- Smoked paprika (.5 tea)
- Cumin (.5 tea)
- Chili powder (.5 tea)
- Olive oil (.5 T)
- Sweet potato (2 medium)

Tools

- Cookie sheet
- Parchment paper
- Veggie knife

Serves: 4

Per Serving (1/4): 19g, 3g, 29g = 76 + 12 + 261 = 349 calories

Directions:

1. Set oven to 400 degrees, and line cookie sheet with parchment paper.

2. Wash and scrub sweet potatoes. Pat dry and cut in half, and cut the halves in half again. Further cut into wedges of 3-4, similar to thick steak fries.

3. Arrange the wedges on a cookie sheet and drizzle with olive oil and sprinkle with paprika, chili powder, salt, and pepper.

4. Place in the oven and roast until the wedges have browned (35-40 minutes). The outside should be crisp, and the inside should be fork tender. Remove from the oven and let cool for 5 minutes. Serve with runny tahini.

Leftovers keep up to five days in the refrigerator (store tahini separately).

2. Creamy Parfait With Berries

~ A bite of lemon cheesecake without the guilt ~

Ingredients

- Poppy seeds (1 tea)
- Almonds, slivered or chopped (1 T)
- Fresh berries - your choice (.25 c)
- Lemon zest (.5 tea)
- Ricotta (.25 c)
- Greek yogurt (.75 c)
- Vanilla extract (dash)

Tools

- Stainless bowl (small)
- Zester
- Veggie knife (chop nuts)
- Ramekins (2 small)

Serves: 2 (.5 cup snacks)

Per Serving (1/2): 11g, 10g, 6g = 44 + 40 + 54 = 138 calories

Directions:

1. Combine ricotta, yogurt, zest, and vanilla in a bowl. If the taste is too sharp, add .25 teaspoon stevia or 1 teaspoon honey.

2. Spoon equal portions into small ramekins and top with berries, nuts, and poppy seeds. Or, use small, reusable containers with berries on top. Put nuts and seeds in a Ziploc bag and put the finishing touches. This makes a great mid-afternoon snack.

3. Savory Oasis Delights

~ Dates, raisins, & pistachios ~

Ingredients

- Fresh ground pepper (.25 tea)
- Ground fennel seeds (1 tea)
- Golden raisins (1 c)
- Pistachios, raw, unsalted, and shelled (1 c)
- Dates, pitted whole (2 c)

Tools

- Food processor
- Measuring cups and spoons

Yield: 32 1-tablespoon date bites

Per Serving (1 tablespoon): 12g, 1g, 1g = 48 + 4 + 9 = 61 calories

Directions:

1. In a food processor, combine and process raisins, pistachios, dates, fennel, and pepper until finely chopped.

2. With a tablespoon, form 32 balls. Store in an airtight container for up to 2 hours at room temperature or refrigerate for later use.

These date bites make a great addition to a cheese board.

4. Pecan Granola

~ A burst of pecan pie in every bite ~

Ingredients

- Sea salt (pinch)
- Cinnamon (.75 tea)
- Safflower oil or melted coconut oil (2 T)
- Pecan pieces (.5 c)
- Brown sugar (.25 c)
- Maple syrup (.5 c)
- Old-fashioned rolled oats (2 c)

Tools

- Cookie sheet (sprayed with cooking spray)
- Stainless bowl (large)
- Measuring cup and spoons

Yield: 2.5 cups

Per Serving (.5 cup): 51g, 5g, 10g = 204 + 20 + 90 = 314 calories

Directions:

1. Set oven to 300 degrees, and prepare a cookie sheet with cooking spray.

2. Add brown sugar, pecans, cinnamon, and salt to the oats. Mix well.

3. Stir in oil and maple syrup and mix well until oats are coated evenly.

4. Pour onto a baking sheet and spread out evenly. Bake for 1 hour. Stir mixture every quarter of an hour so that nothing burns.

5. Cool completely before storing in an airtight container. If granola is still warm when stored, the condensation that builds up will cause the granola to get limp and soft.

5. Jumpin' Quinoa Munch Bars

~ Chocolate & peanut butter crunch bars ~

Ingredients

- PB2 or ground almond flour (2.5 T + 1 T)
- Almond extract (a drop) - if using almond flour
- Water (2 T)
- Vanilla extract (.5 tea)
- Quinoa, dry (1 c)
- Semi-sweet chocolate bars (4 4-oz Baker's)

Tools

- Heavy-bottom saucepan (medium)
- Stainless bowl (medium and small)
- Cookie sheet with parchment paper

Yields: 20 bars

Per Serving (1/20): 12g, 2g, 4g = 48 + 8 + 36 = 92 calories

Directions:

1. Heat pan over medium-high heat. Pour in a quarter of your quinoa, swirling the pan occasionally. You should hear the grain start to pop like popcorn. It will start slow then pick up a fairly steady popping pattern, then slow down again. Continue to swirl pan while popping to

avoid burning the grain. Remove from heat when the popping slows. You don't want the grain to get darker than golden brown. Transfer toasted grain to a small bowl and repeat three more times.

2. Melt your chocolate in a small bowl in the microwave or over a double boiler.

3. In a medium bowl, combine and stir well the quinoa, 1 tablespoon PB2 or almond flour, chocolate, and vanilla.

4. Spread the chocolate mixture on a cookie sheet prepared with parchment paper. Don't try to spread to edge of the sheet but into a square or rectangular shape until the mixture is about .5 inches thick.

5. In a small bowl, whisk together PB2 (or almond flour and almond extract) and water. Drizzle over the chocolate slab and refrigerate for 2 hours.

6. Cut into 2o squares and store in an airtight container in the refrigerator. I keep them on the parchment when layering so that the bars don't stick to each other.

6. Evening Pick-Me-Up

~ Mini cheese board ~

Ingredients

- Almonds, toasted (1 c)
- Cheddar cheese, sliced (4 oz)

Tools

- Paper towel
- Paring knife

Serves: 4

Per Serving (1/4): 6g, 12g, 21g = 24 + 48 + 189 = 261 calories

Directions:

1. Place nuts on a paper towel in the microwave and zap for 1.5 minutes. Remove from the oven and cool.

2. Slice about 1 inch of the cheese brick, and divide that into four pieces. Repeat this until you have 4 servings of cheese.

3. Place 1/4 nuts and 1 oz (4 pieces) of cheese on each plate and serve.

7. Savory Herb Roasted Potatoes

~ Rosemary & thyme ~

Ingredients

- Parsley, chopped (2 tea)
- Red potatoes, quartered (1.25 lb)
- Sea salt and fresh ground pepper (to taste)
- Fresh thyme, chopped (1 T)
- Fresh rosemary, chopped (1 T)
- Olive oil (1 T)

Tools

- Stainless bowl (medium)
- Veggie knife
- Teaspoons
- Cutting board
- Baking sheet
- Cooking spray

Serves: 4

Per Serving (1/4): 23g, 3g, 4g = 92 + 12 + 36 = 140 calories

Directions:

1. Set oven to 425 degrees. Scrub potatoes, pat dry, and cut into even-sized wedges. Transfer to mixing bowl.

2. Chop thyme and rosemary, and add them to the potatoes. Add salt and pepper, drizzle olive oil, and mix well until all pieces are coated.

3. Prepare a baking sheet with cooking spray and evenly spread the potatoes over the pan.

4. Place the pan in the oven and bake for 30 minutes (stirring once). Potatoes should be fork-tender and golden brown.

5. Remove from the oven and transfer to a serving platter.

8. Side Salad

~ Dress it up any way you want ~

Ingredients

- Mixed greens (4 c)
- Carrot, grated (1 medium)
- Celery, chopped (1 stalk)
- Green olive, Greek olive (1 each)
- Grape tomatoes, halved (.5 c)

Tools

- Veggie knife
- Grater
- Chopping board
- Stainless bowl (large)

Serves: 4

Per Serving (1/4): 3g, 1g, .5g = 12 + 4 + 4.5 = 20.5 calories

Directions:

1. Combine mixed greens, carrots, celery, and tomatoes in mixing bowl and toss well.

2. Divide evenly into salad bowls and top with 2 olives per bowl.

3. Serve with your choice of dressing.

9. Good Fat Snack

~ *A lite bite* ~

Ingredients

- Walnuts, toasted (.25c)
- Hard-boiled egg (1)
- Sea salt (to taste)

Tools

- Paper towel

Serves: 1

Per Serving (1): 3g, 13g, 23g = 12 + 52 + 207 = 271 calories

Directions:

1. Place nuts on a paper towel in the microwave and zap for 1.5 minutes. Remove from oven and let cool.

3. Place nuts and on a plate and serve with a pinch of salt.

10. Power Snack

~ Kills cravings every time ~

Ingredients

- Hard-boiled egg (2)
- Sea salt (to taste)

Tools

- Paper towel

Serves: 1

Per Serving (1): 1g, 11g, 9g = 4 + 44 + 81 = 129 calories

Directions:

1. Serve eggs with a pinch of salt.

11. Sun-Kissed Quinoa

~ Sun-dried tomatoes & spinach ~

Ingredients

- Feta cheese, crumbled (.5 c)
- Sun-dried tomatoes, chopped (3 T)
- Lemon juice (1 T)
- Sea salt and fresh ground pepper (to taste)
- Water (2 c)
- Quinoa (1 c)
- Spinach, chopped (2 c)
- Garlic, minced (4 cloves)
- Onion, diced (1 medium)
- Safflower oil (1 T)

Tools

- Nonstick skillet (large)
- Saucepan (medium)
- Veggie knife
- Measuring cups and spoons

Serves: 6

Per Serving (1/6): 22g, 7g, 7g = 88 + 28 + 63 = 179 calories

Directions:

1. Using oiled skillet, saute onion and garlic over medium heat until onions begin to caramelize. Add spinach and allow to wilt, then stir into the onion mixture.

2. Add quinoa and water to the saucepan and bring to a boil on high heat. Turn the heat down to medium-low and simmer for about 15 minutes or until the water is absorbed.

3. Stir in tomatoes, lemon juice, and feta cheese to the quinoa mixture and season to taste. Serve warm or cold. It can be stored in an airtight container for up to five days.

12. Steamed Asparagus

~ Doesn't get much easier or tastier ~

Ingredients

- Water (.75 c)
- Sea salt (.25 tea)
- Butter (1 tea)
- Asparagus (1 bunch)

Tools

- Saucepan (medium)

Serves: 4

Per Serving (1/4): 3g, 2g, 1g = 12 + 8 + 9 = 29 calories

Directions:

1. Rinse and snap ends off the asparagus spears (the spears will naturally break at the point where the fibers become tough).

2. Place in a pan (snap in half if they don't lay flat), and add water over medium-high heat. Add a pinch of salt and cover with a lid (set timer for 5 minutes). The spears are done when they are fork-tender. Although, I like mine with a little resistance, so I take them off before they are fork-tender.

3. Spread butter and serve warm.

13. Kale

~ *Soy sauce, lemon juice, garlic* ~

Ingredients

- Sea salt and fresh ground pepper (to taste)
- Soy sauce (1 tea)
- Garlic, minced (1 T)
- Olive oil (1 T)
- Lemon juice (2 T)
- Water (1.5 c)
- Kale, chopped (12 c)

Tools

- Saucepan (large)
- Stainless bowl (small)
- Fork for whisking
- Chopping board
- Veggie knife
- Measuring spoons

Serves: 6

Per Serving (1/6): 1g, 1g, 2g = 44 + 20 + 117 calories

Directions:

1. Rinse kale in a colander, drain thoroughly, and chop coarsely.

2. In a large pan, add water, kale, salt, and pepper, to taste over high heat. Cover with lid and set a timer for 8-10 minutes until tender. Remove kale from the heat and drain in a colander. Return to pan.

3. In a small bowl, add soy sauce, garlic, olive oil, and lemon juice, and whisk them together with a fork. Drizzle dressing over the kale and toss until evenly distributed.

14. Orzo Salad

~ Orzo tossed in red wine dressing ~

Ingredients

- Feta cheese, crumbled (.5 c)
- Greek olives, halved (12)
- Cucumber, chopped (1 medium)
- Grape tomatoes, halved (1 c)
- Sea salt and fresh ground pepper (to taste)
- Sugar (.5 tea)
- Dried oregano (1.5 tea)
- Red wine vinegar (.3 c)
- Fresh parsley (.5 c)
- Red onion, finely chopped (1 medium)
- Olive oil (4 T)
- Orzo pasta, uncooked (1 c)

Tools

- Saucepan (medium)
- Large bowl
- Veggie knife
- Chopping board
- Whisk
- Measuring cups and spoons

Serves: 4

Per Serving (1/4): 13g, 5g, 11g = 52 + 20 + 99 = 171 calories

Directions:

1. Prepare pasta according to instructions on the package. Drain, add 2 tablespoons of olive oil, mix well, and set aside.

2. In a large bowl, combine vinegar oregano, salt, sugar, pepper, parsley, onion, and the remaining 2 tablespoons of olive oil. Whisk ingredients together, add pasta, and mix well until orzo is coated with dressing.

3. Cover and refrigerate for at least 2 and up to 24 hours. Before serving, fold in tomatoes, cucumber, olives, and cheese.

15. Cuc & Dill Salad

~Look, no lettuce, Mom! ~

Ingredients

- Feta, crumbled (.25 c)
- Fresh dill, chopped (1 T)
- Red onion, sliced thin (half onion)
- Cucumbers, peeled, halved, seeded, and thinly sliced (1.75 c)
- Sea salt and fresh ground pepper (to taste)
- Dried oregano (1 tea)
- Olive oil (2 T)
- Red wine vinegar (3 T)

Tools

- Veggie knife
- Stainless bowl (medium)
- Wisk
- Chopping board
- Measuring cups and spoons

Serves: 4

Per Serving (1/4): 4g, 2g, 9g = 16 + 8 + 81 = 105 calories

Directions:

1. In a bowl, combine vinegar, salt, pepper, oregano and whisk in olive oil.

2. Add dill, onion, cucumbers, and feta to the dressing. Toss to coat cucumbers well. Taste before serving, and adjust seasoning as needed.

16. The Greek Beat Salad

~Beets, feta, & mint ~

Ingredients

- Red wine vinegar (2 T)
- Olive oil (3 T)
- Sea salt and fresh ground pepper (to taste)
- Ground coriander (1 tea)
- Fresh parsley, chopped (1 T)
- Fresh basil, julienned (2 T)
- Fresh mint (2 T)
- Feta cheese, crumbled (.25 c)
- Garlic, minced very, very fine (2 T)
- Beets, chopped (2 large - about 4 c)

Tools

- Saucepan (medium)
- Veggie knife
- Chopping board
- Measuring spoons
- Stainless bowl (large)

Serves: 6

Per Serving (1/6): 7g, 2g, 9g = 28 + 8 + 81 = 117 calories

Directions:

1. Boil beets over medium-high heat for 1 hour or until they are fork-tender. Remove from the heat, and let it cool.

2. Slice, chop, or dice beets as you like and transfer into a mixing bowl. Add the rest of the ingredients and fold in gently until the beets are coated. Serve and enjoy.

17. Mediterranean Quinoa Fritters

~ Cheesy, garlicky with zucchini ~

Ingredients

- Olive oil (3 T)
- Sea salt and fresh ground pepper (to taste)
- Panko crumbs (1 cup)
- Parmigiana-Reggiano cheese, grated (1 cup)
- Dried oregano (.25 tea)
- Garlic, minced (3 cloves)
- Egg (1)
- Quinoa, dry (.5 c)
- Water (1 c)
- Sea salt (.5 tea)
- Zucchini, grated (2 c)

Tools

- Cast iron skillet (large)
- Colander
- Saucepan (medium)
- Measuring cups and spoons

Yields: 14 fritters

Per Serving (1 fritter): 7g, 7g, 7g = 28 + 28 + 63 = 119 calories

Directions:

1. Grate zucchini using a box grater, and place it in a colander with .5 teaspoons of salt and mix. This will help draw some of the moist from the zucchini. After 10 minutes, dry zucchini with a paper towel and place in a large bowl.

2. While the zucchini is sweating, cook quinoa by adding quinoa and water in the saucepan and bring to boil over high heat. Reduce heat to medium-low and finish cooking for 10 minutes. Remove from heat, stir, and let stand for 10 minutes or more.

3. Add garlic, oregano, cheese, panko, egg, and seasoning. Mix together thoroughly.

4. While oil and skillet are heating over medium to medium-high heat, shape the mixture into 2-3 inch patties.

5. In batches of 3 or 4, place patties in a skillet and cook until golden for about 4 minutes each side. As fritters are done, transfer to a plate lined with a paper towel to absorb excess oil.

6. Serve hot with your favorite dipping sauce or yogurt, soy sauce, or sour cream.

Chapter 10: Shopping Guide and Food List

Foods to Eat:
- *Lean meats*: fish, seafood, vegetables, fruits, nuts, whole grains, herbs, spices, olive oil, and safflower oil
- *Use moderately*: poultry, natural nut butters, eggs, low-fat dairy, and wine
- *Use sparingly*: red meat, butter, whole milk, higher-fat dairy, bacon, and sausage
- *Pass on*: trans fat (hydrogenated fat)

Pantry List:
- Olive oil
- Quinoa
- Honey
- Soy sauce
- Sea salt
- Black peppercorns
- Quinoa
- Greek olives
- Canned: garbanzo beans and beets
- Dried or ground: cumin, thyme, oregano, cinnamon, paprika, red pepper flakes, and dill weed
- Baking powder and baking soda
- Mayonnaise and stone-ground mustard
- Whole grain flour

Fresh List:
- Skim milk
- Feta cheese
- Non-homogenized yogurt
- Whole grain bread
- Garlic
- Yellow onions
- Green onions
- Mixed greens
- Carrots
- Celery
- Fresh basil and mint
- Eggs
- Protein for immediate use

Chapter 11: Charting Your Success

Weight/Macro Chart

Using a macro calculator from one of the websites listed below or a recommendation from your physician, you can enter your body specifications and record your goal numbers.

Enter: sex, age, weight, height, and degree of exercise/job type

Record: grams per day, grams per meal, calories per day, calories per meal, calories to maintain current weight, calories for fat loss, and calories for extreme fat loss.

Set Up Your Goal

- Decide what fits your schedule.
- Will you be able to add some exercise as well as cut calories to reach your goal faster?
- Will you reduce your intake of processed foods by increasing the number of home-cooked meals per week?
- Will you make better choices when eating out?
- Record what you eat. Only you can hold yourself accountable.
- Stay away from the scale, and stick with your plan.

Make Your Meal Plan

Date:

Breakfast		gCarbs	gProt	gFat		cCarbs	cProt	cFat	Calories
Snack									
Lunch									
Snack									
Dinner									
Snack									
Daily Totals									

Exercise Chart

If you are not using a tool such as myfitnesspal, a simple chart will do. It's all about accountability.

Example entries:

9/9/99, 4:30 p.m., 4:50 p.m., Dog Walk, Moderate (if it's a stop and sniff day - Low)

9/9/99, 6:30 p.m., 8:00 p.m., Basketball, High

Exercise for Week:				
Date	Start	End	Type	Intensity

Recipe Macro/Calorie Table

Breakfast	Portion	gCarbs	gProt	gFat	cCarbs	cProt	cFat	Calories
Basted Egg with Smoked Salmon on Toast	1	28	13	19	112	52	171	335
Breakfast Casserole for Eight	1/8	36	15	15	144	60	135	339
Almond Ricotta Spread with Fruit	1/6	31	9	10	124	36	90	250
Savory Egg Cups with Goat Cheese	2 cups	5	14	11	20	56	99	175
Sunny Breakfast Salad	1/4	19	12	16	76	48	144	268
Berry Breakfast Quinoa	1/4	54	12	8	216	48	72	336
Caramelized Onion Egg Skillet	1/6	20	12	13	80	48	117	245
Rosemary & Spinach Frittata	1/8	5	10	10	20	40	90	150
Whole Wheat Pancakes with Greek Yogurt	2 cakes	31	10	9	124	40	81	245

MEAL PLANNING FOR BEGINNERS

Topping								
Homemade Whole Wheat Pancake Mix	1/10	73	10	24	292	40	216	548
Feta, Quinoa, Egg Muffin	2 muffins	12	13	15	48	52	135	235

Lunch	Portion	gCarbs	gProt	gFat	cCarbs	cProt	cFat	Calories
Shrimp Salad	1/4	16	30	15	64	120	135	319
Tropical Salad: Fruit, Nuts & More	1/4	23	21	28	92	84	252	428
Greek Salad	1/4	25	39	23	100	156	207	463
Garbanzo Lettuce Wrap	1/4	58	14	6	232	56	54	342
Shrimp Sandwich with Bleu Cheese Dressing	1/4	60	43	26	240	172	234	646
Citrus Pesto Chicken Salad	1/6	4	25	5	16	100	45	161
Pan Bagna	1/6	52	20	20	208	80	180	468
Tuna Salad	1/4	2	12	5	8	48	45	101
Dilled Chicken on Quinoa	1/4	18	30	23	72	120	207	399
Creamy Chicken Salad with Basil Pesto	1/6	6	21	22	24	84	198	306
Picnic Plate	1/4	57	14	15	228	56	135	419
Beet Hummus	1/10	29	10	6	116	40	54	210
Hummus	1/4 cup	27	8	10	108	32	90	230
Tabbouleh	1/4	20	4	8	80	16	72	168
Balsamic Vinaigrette	1 T	0.2	0	3	0.8	0	27	27.8
Pine Nut Pesto	1 T	0	1	6	0	4	54	58
Lemon Tahini Dressing	1 T	2	1	7	8	4	63	75
Lemon Mustard Dressing	1 T	1	0	2	4	0	18	22

MEAL PLANNING FOR BEGINNERS

Bleu Cheese Dressing	1 T	1	1	6	4	4	54	62
Citrus Pesto	1 T	4	1	0	16	4	0	20
Herb Veggie Spread	1/4 cup	9	6	5	36	24	45	105
Yogurt Cheese	1 cup	24	24	8	96	96	72	264
Potato Salad	1/8	20	5	8	80	20	72	172
Poppy Seed Dressing	1 T	6	0	9	24	0	81	105
Red Wine Vinaigrette	1 T	0.5	0	3	2	0	27	29

Dinner	Portion	gCarbs	gProt	gFat	cCarbs	cProt	cFat	Calories
Baked Falafel	1/4	29	8	9	116	32	81	229
Lime Grilled Pork Tenderloin	1/6	2	40	12	8	160	108	276
Greek Lemon Chicken with Herb Rice	1/5	31	7	15	124	28	135	287
Stuffed Onions	1/6	35	26	29	140	104	261	505
Greek-Style Grouper	1/4	0	42	9	0	168	81	249
Broiled Snapper	1/4	0	45	6	0	180	54	234
Pan-Broiled Chicken Breast	1/4	0	71	15	0	284	135	419
Grilled Lamb & Fig Kebabs	1/8	40	58	21	160	232	189	581
Chicken Pitas	1/4	9	92	31	36	368	279	683
Mediterranean Shrimp Fajitas	1/4	35	43	10	140	172	90	402
Spicy Pan-Seared Salmon	1/4	0	33	17	0	132	153	285
Greek Flank Steak	1/6	1	43	21	4	172	189	365
Mediterranean Stuffed Peppers	1/6	35	19	6	140	76	54	270
Arugula Shrimp Salad with White Beans	1/4	23	34	9	92	136	81	309

	Portion	gCarbs	gProt	gFat	cCarbs	cProt	cFat	Calories
Quick Mediterranean Chicken Pasta	1/6	34	19	13	136	76	117	329
Baked Greek Salmon in a Pouch	1/4	9	40	28	36	160	252	448
Tzatziki	1/6	3	2	0.5	12	8	4.5	24.5
Toasty Couscous	1/4	34	6	4	136	24	36	196
Salsa Fresca	1/4	6	1	1	24	4	9	37

Desserts	Portion	gCarbs	gProt	gFat	cCarbs	cProt	cFat	Calories
Vegan No-Bake Cookies	1 cookie	8	3	7	32	12	63	107
Yogurt Cheese Cake	1/10	15	6	3	60	24	27	111
Luscious Baked Pears	1/4	86	8	20	344	32	180	556
Funky Monkey Yogurt	1/8	29	23	33	116	92	297	505
Raspberry Cream Cups	1 cup	25	4	25	100	16	225	341
Grecian Cinnamon Apple Cake	1/12	50	7	23	200	28	207	435
Mediterranean Mousse	1/4	28	9	10	112	36	90	238

Snacks	Portion	gCarbs	gProt	gFat	cCarbs	cProt	cFat	Calories
Sweet Potatoes with Sesame Sauce	1/4	19	3	29	76	12	261	349
Creamy Parfait with Berries	1/2	11	10	6	44	40	54	138
Savory Oasis Delights	1 T	12	1	1	48	4	9	61
Pecan Granola	1/2 cup	51	5	10	204	20	90	314
Jumpin' Quinoa Munch Bars	1 Bar	12	2	4	48	8	36	92
Evening Pick-Me-Up	1/4	6	12	21	24	48	189	261

MEAL PLANNING FOR BEGINNERS

Savory Herb Roasted Potatoes	1/4	23	3	4		92	12	36	140
Side Salad	1/4	3	1	0.5		12	4	4.5	20.5
Good Fat Snack	1	3	13	23		12	52	207	271
Power Snack	1	1	11	9		4	44	81	129
Sun-Kissed Quinoa	1/6	22	7	7		88	28	63	179
Steamed Asparagus	1/4	3	2	1		12	8	9	29
Kale	1/6	1	1	2		4	4	18	26
Orzo Salad	1/4	13	5	11		52	20	99	171
Cuc & Dill Salad	1/4	4	2	9		16	8	81	105
Beet Salad	1/6	7	2	9		28	8	81	117
Mediterranean Quinoa Fritters	1/14	7	7	7		28	28	63	119
Protein Drink	1	4	20	2		16	80	18	114

MEAL PLANNING FOR BEGINNERS

Online Resources

- *www.myfitnesspal.com* is an excellent health and fitness site to help figure out macro numbers in the food you eat. The site will also help you track food, water, and exercise to help you reach your health and fitness goals.
- www.freedieting.com has a variety of tools and calculators. I used the Daily Calorie Needs calculator to figure out the Maintenance, Moderate, and Extreme calorie totals. It also has information on diet and exercise that you might find beneficial.
- www.bodybuilding.com also has a macro calculator.
- www.verywellfit.com has a recipe calculator to help you figure out the macros in your favorite recipes. It can be a little persnickety with the descriptions, so make sure you enter a plain description. For example: "*1 cup potatoes, chopped*" is fine, but "*1 cup Idaho potatoes, steamed, peeled*" is going to make it go into a loop trying to parse all the terminology.

Conclusion

Thank you for making it to the end of *Meal Planning for Beginners*. Let's hope it was informative and able to provide you with all of the tools you need to achieve your goals whatever they may be.

The next step is to put your plan into action. That plan is all about taking good care of yourself. Make small changes and build confidence in your ability to reach that goal. This important step in your life is about the journey, not the result. If you are cooking for or with family members, involve them in the meal planning, shopping, and cooking.

Don't set hard, fast deadlines for losing x pounds in x weeks. Instead, concentrate on enriching other aspects of your life. Are you bored in walking the same old blocks? Take a stroll around your downtown or in other neighborhoods. We have a group that walks a different park every weekend. How many city, county, and state parks do you have in your area? This is also a great way to reconnect the family once a week.

Join a new club: bicycling, painting, gardening, or whatever you like to do or always wanted to try. Take a class: yoga, drawing, or pet obedience. Volunteer. You see, you didn't just get a book on meal planning; you got a book on life planning. You want something better, then go and get it.

Finally, if you found this book useful in any way, a review on Amazon is always appreciated!

Made in the USA
Monee, IL
12 June 2020